Generalized Dermatitis
in Clinical Practice

Susan T. Nedorost

Generalized Dermatitis in Clinical Practice

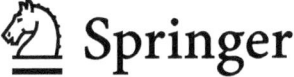 Springer

Susan T. Nedorost
University Hospitals Case
Medical Center
UHMG Dermatology
Ohio
USA

ISBN 978-1-4471-2896-0   ISBN 978-1-4471-2897-7   (eBook)
DOI 10.1007/978-1-4471-2897-7
Springer Dordrecht Heidelberg New York London

Library of Congress Control Number: 2012942606

Printed on acid-free paper

Springer is part of Springer Science+Business Media (www.springer.com)

Dedicated to my husband Bob, my anchor who supports my passion for learning from my patients and my colleagues

Preface

Ideal dermatitis care is patient centered and includes critical thinking about the unique genetic and environmental factors that influence the patient's symptoms.

Like other complex medical disease, dermatitis care occurs in a time-pressured ambulatory care system that is, at times, fragmented. When patients visit a dermatologist, they present a multifactorial disease for which basic research has not fully elucidated the pathophysiology. This is in contrast to other dermatological diagnoses such as skin cancer, where a reliable diagnosis and treatment plan can often be formulated within a few minutes.

Dermatitis challenges clinicians to problem-solve for our patients, to combine our resources across disciplines, and to apply our knowledge to public health prevention.

Our patients are our partners and our teachers as we aim to improve care for this common and burdensome condition.

Susan T. Nedorost

Acknowledgments

Interdisciplinary Care: The members of our Interdisciplinary Eczema Clinic lkjtelk were critical to developing the concepts of interdisciplinary care in Chap. 11, as well as honing concepts regarding atopic dermatitis.

The University Hospitals Case Medical Center Interdisciplinary Eczema Clinic

Howard Hall Ph.D. – behavioral psychology

Nicole Lidyard RD – dietetics

Elizabeth Marteny RN – dermatology nurse

Suwimon Pootangkum M.D. – dermatitis research fellow

Eli Silver M.D. – allergy/immunology

Dermatology residents Ligaya Park DO and others

And former founding members:

Mary Smith RN CNS – clinical nurse specialist

Joan Tamburro DO – pediatric dermatology

Hypereosinophilic Syndrome: contributors – Min Deng, B.S.; Peggy Myung, M.D.; Alvin H. Schmaier M.D.

Diagnosis of Generalized Dermatitis: contributors: Suzanne Smith D.O., Tamila Kindwall-Keller D.O., and Hillard Lazarus M.D.

Glossary contributor: Suwimon Pootangkum M.D., Kord Honda M.D. contributed the photomicrographs

I also appreciate the support of the University Hospital Case Medical Center Dermatology chairman Kevin D. Cooper M.D.

Contents

Chapter 1
Introduction

Some forms of dermatitis are very mild and self-limited, but for patients with generalized disease, the burden is great (Fig. 1.1).

Quality of life suffers due to the symptom of itch interfering with sleep and concentration. Lost time from school and work and numerous topical and systemic therapies are costly.

Despite a burden of disease equal to many other common, chronic diseases, public awareness and research attention have been insufficient.

Generalized dermatitis is poorly characterized and imprecisely treated for several reasons.

Problems with the Definition

This is in part due to the inconsistent definition of dermatitis. Even among dermatologists, the term can be used to denote only atopic skin disease or a broader range of inflammatory skin disease [1]. Some even include papulosquamous diseases in the dermatitis category.

Definition of the term eczema is also imprecise. Some investigators prefer the term eczema because it is better recognized by patients, and patient perspective is an important part of outcomes research [2]. However, terms like atopic eczema can imply mechanism that is not intended; specifically, allergists may over-utilize serum IgE testing in an attempt to

S.T. Nedorost, *Generalized Dermatitis in Clinical Practice,*
DOI 10.1007/978-1-4471-2897-7_1,
© Springer-Verlag London 2012

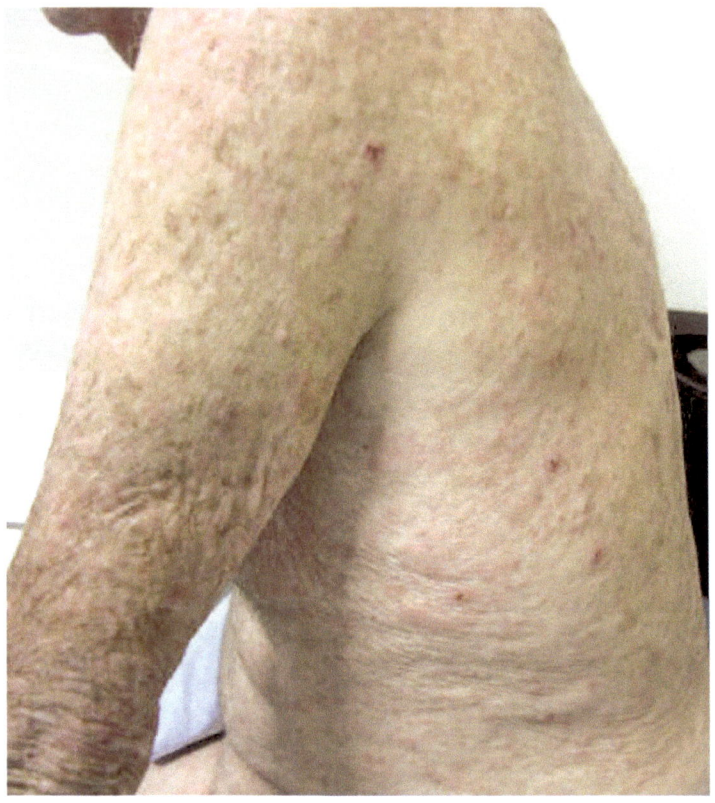

FIGURE 1.1 Chronic severe generalized dermatitis

support a diagnosis of atopic eczema when these tests are not specific for any sub-type of dermatitis and are not required for diagnosis [3].

In this work, dermatitis and eczema are used interchangeably to denote the entire spectrum of disease.

Problems with the Diagnosis and Treatment

Beyond the problem of the definition, dermatitis is almost always multi-factorial. Most patients have some irritant dermatitis in combination with either atopic, allergic contact, stasis, or

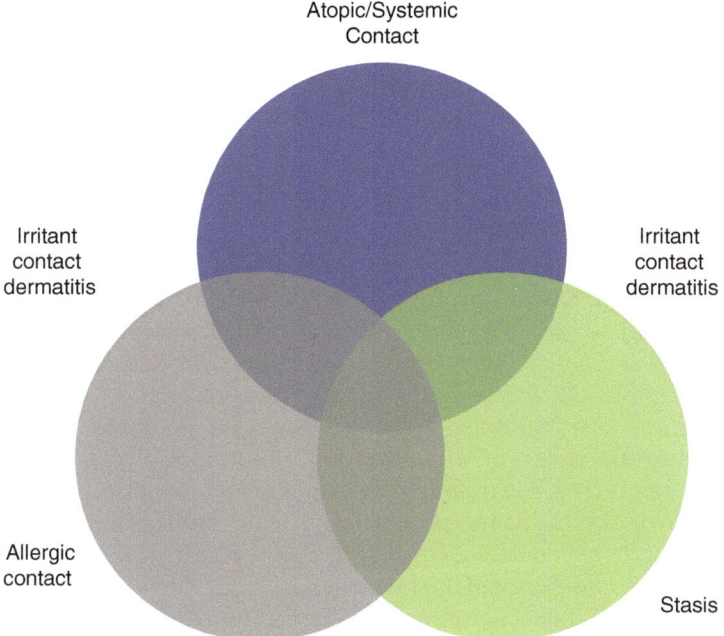

FIGURE 1.2 Clinical and basic science research requires clear definition of dermatitis cohorts

systemic contact dermatitis. This greatly increases the difficulty of creating a similar cohort of patients for research (Fig. 1.2)

Treatment of chronic dermatitis requires attention to barrier repair, allergic triggers, and infection. Without concurrent management of each of these factors, solitary interventions usually fail.

The need to identify multiple diagnostic subtypes and to manage more than one therapeutic approach often overwhelms both physicians and patients. In North America, the most common, simplest form of acute generalized contact dermatitis results from skin exposure to poison ivy. This is appropriately treated with systemic corticosteroids for 2–3 weeks, and no other intervention is required. However, all other types of generalized dermatitis require multiple diagnostic and therapeutic interventions. Topical and systemic corticosteroids are never appropriate as mono-therapy for chronic dermatitis, but are commonly used in this fashion.

Problems with the Care Team

In the United States, patients with generalized dermatitis may seek care from primary care providers, urgent care or emergency settings, allergists, and/or dermatologists.

Government agencies also interface with dermatitis. For example, the Bureau of Worker's Compensation is involved in occupational cases, and the Women Infants and Children nutrition program with selection of formulae for pediatric patients. There is usually poor communication between these providers and agencies which results in conflicting messages to patients.

An international Delphi exercise including patient perspective, clinicians, journal editors, and one regulatory agency outlined core measures to be included in outcomes research: physician scoring of physical exam (e.g. Severity Scoring of Atopic Dermatitis [SCORAD] or Eczema Area and Severity Index {EASI}), symptoms, and long-term control of flares. The type of eczema studied in this project appeared to be atopic eczema (dermatitis), but inclusion criteria for patient stakeholders other than belonging to an advocacy or support group was not specifically stated [4].

Aim of This Work

Increased research focus and combined interdisciplinary attention to dermatitis will brighten the future for patients. This monograph utilizes scientific literature to guide classification and treatment of generalized dermatitis without losing site of the clinical reality that many of our most complicated patients have more than one inflammatory skin

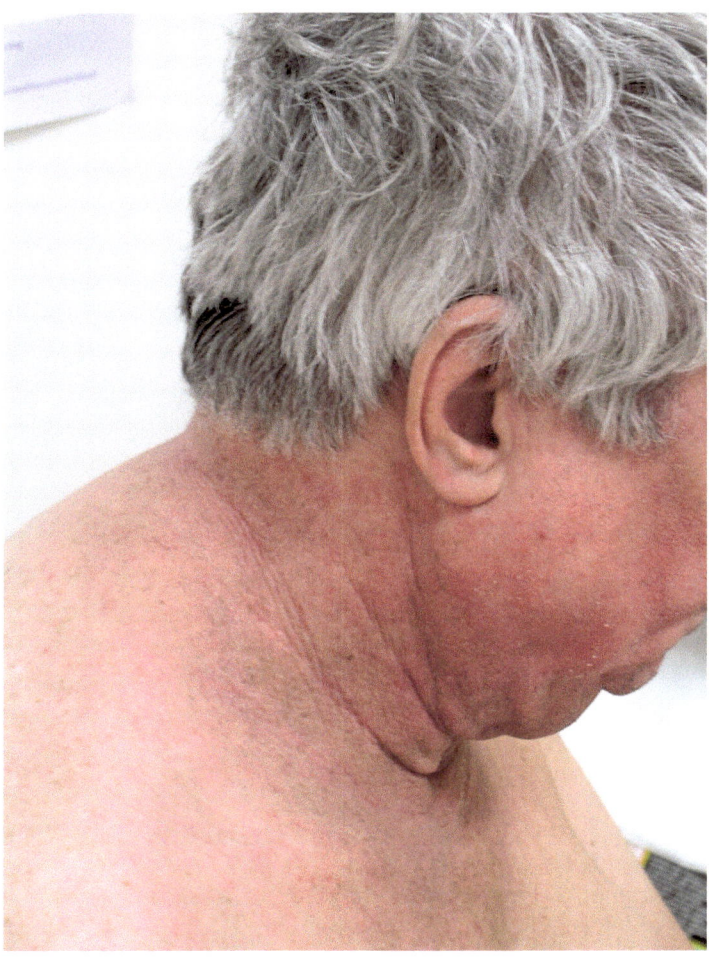

FIGURE 1.3 Generalized atopic dermatitis/systemic contact dermatitis (patch tests positive vanillin and eugenol, negative to Balsam of Peru)

disease (Fig. 1.3) and that other inflammatory dermatoses may mimic generalized dermatitis (Fig. 1.4).

Interdisciplinary communication depends on reducing specialty-specific jargon; a glossary of dermatological and immunological terms is included to this end.

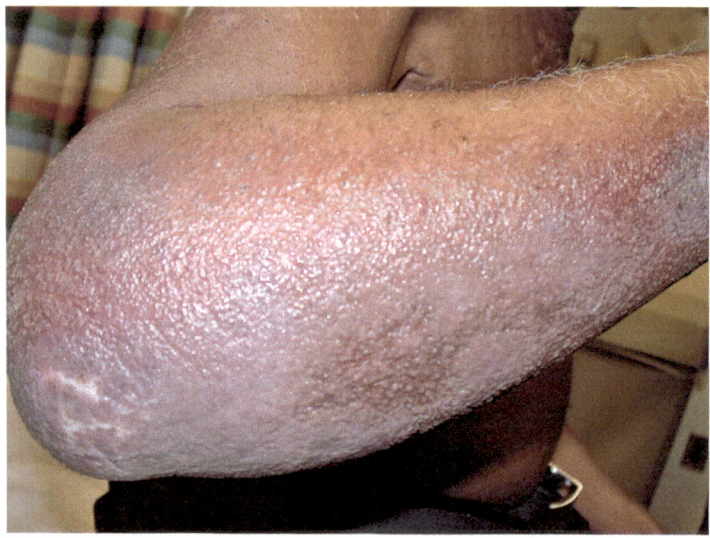

Figure 1.4 Drug eruption in a patient with psoriasis. Note the underlying sharply demarcated (psoriatic) plaques. The superimposed papules represent a dermal hypersensitivity reaction to a medication, but the superimposed patterns mimic generalized dermatitis

References

1. Smith SM, Nedorost ST. "Dermatitis" defined. Dermatitis. 2010; 21(5):248–50.
2. Schmitt J, Flohr C, Williams HC. Outcome measures, case definition, and nomenclature are all important and distinct aspects of atopic eczema: a call for harmonization. J Invest Dermatol. 2012;132(2):473–4.
3. Hanifin JM. Atopic dermatitis nomenclature variants can impede harmonization. J Invest Dermatol. 2012;132(2):472–3.
4. Schmitt J, Langan S, Stamm T, Williams HC. Harmonizing Outcome Measurements in Eczema (HOME) Delphi panel. Core outcome domains for controlled trials and clinical record-keeping in eczema: international multiperspective Delphi consensus process. J Invest Dermatol. 2011;131(3):623–30.

Chapter 2
Generalized Dermatitis: The Basics

Key Concepts

- Dermatitis is multi-factorial
- Barrier dysfunction, infection, and immune response are key components
- Inter-disciplinary care including dermatology, allergy, and psychology and specialized nurse education best addresses patient needs

Introduction

This work focuses on generalized dermatitis; that is, dermatitis affecting several anatomical units. Chronic generalized dermatitis is more complex to diagnosis than localized dermatitis because the differential diagnosis includes mimics of dermatitis such as bullous pemphigoid and dermatomyositis. Asking the patient where dermatitis first appeared on the skin can help to direct history taking.

Localized dermatitis such as seborrheic or nummular dermatitis may be sufficiently treated with intermittent use of topical corticosteroids. However, although commonly used for generalized dermatitis, topical corticosteroids are insufficient.

S.T. Nedorost, *Generalized Dermatitis in Clinical Practice,*
DOI 10.1007/978-1-4471-2897-7_2,
© Springer-Verlag London 2012

Precise characterization of the dermatitis allows for more directed and appropriate treatment. The multi-factorial nature of dermatitis has impeded both clinical and basic science research; diagnostic nomenclature is imprecise as discussed in the introduction.

Definition

Dermatitis is the result of environmental and immunological events. Impaired keratinocytes allow fluid to accumulate in the epidermis (spongiosis) (Fig. 2.1). As epidermal barrier function weakens environmental insults trigger the innate and adaptive immune response, and lymphocytes move into the dermis (Fig. 2.2). With chronic inflammation, the epidermis thickens and can appear psoriasiform (Fig. 2.3), but dermatitis is distinct from papulosquamous disorders such as psoriasis and lichen planus.

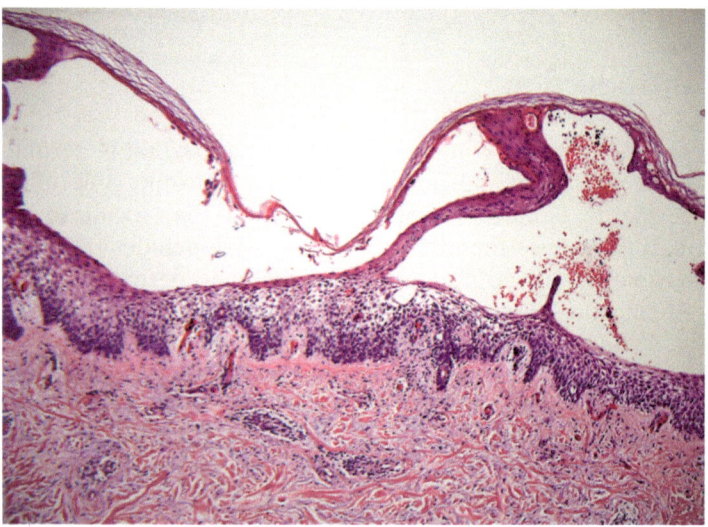

FIGURE 2.1 Histology of acute dermatitis

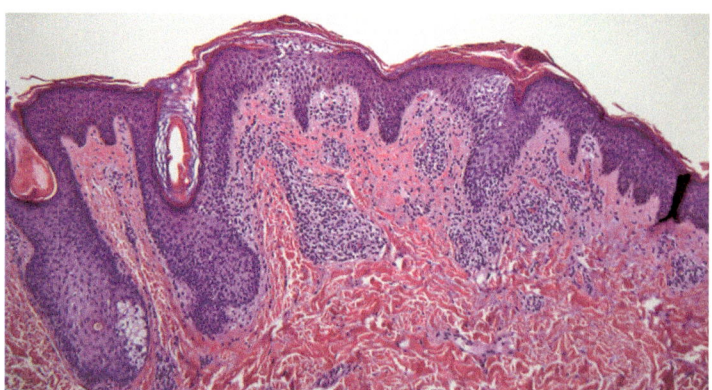

FIGURE 2.2 Histology of subacute dermatitis

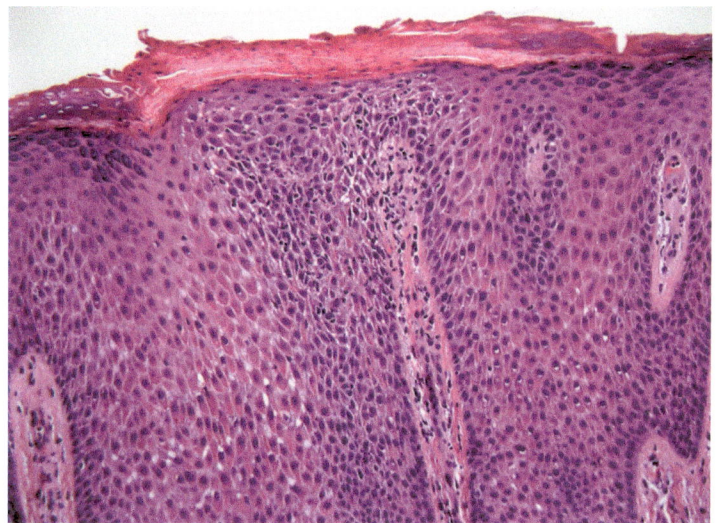

FIGURE 2.3 Histology of chronic dermatitis

Patients experience itch, redness, and changes in the epidermis that foretell the duration of the inflammation. Acute dermatitis is vesicular (Fig. 2.4), while sub-acute and chronic dermatitis result in more thickened epidermis (Fig. 2.5).

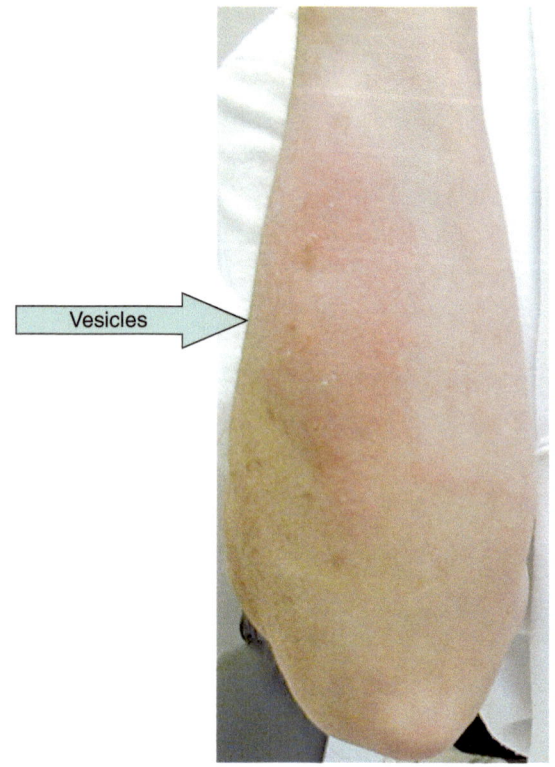

FIGURE 2.4 Acute (poison ivy) dermatitis

Provocation is often multi-factorial, even within individual patients. Chronic friction causes hyperkeratosis that can appear psoriasiform, especially on hands (Fig. 2.6). Secondary infection of fissures and excoriations causes pain that can be more severe than itch.

Pathophysiology

Barrier dysfunction is present in all forms of dermatitis. Genetic differences in genes such as filaggrin in atopic dermatitis can weaken epidermal integrity, and keratinocytes

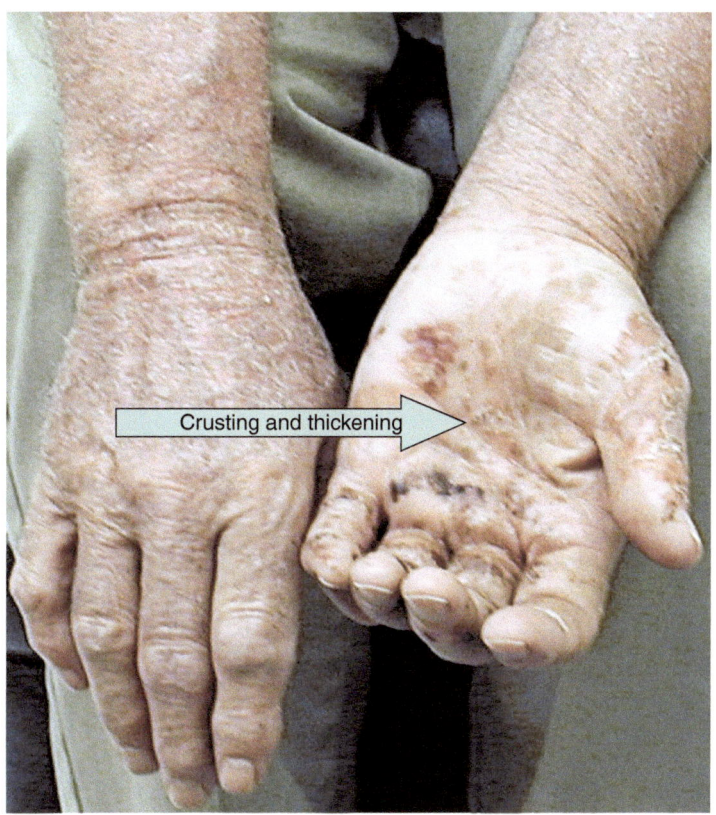

FIGURE 2.5 Subacute dermatitis

produce less filaggrin even without genetic mutation in the presence of Th2 cytokines [1]. In occupational dermatitis, rapid wet/dry cycles due to wet work in low humidity conditions elicits fissures in the epidermis that become inflamed. Aggressive personal hygiene in areas of susceptible skin such as the face, eyelid, and genitalia provokes irritant dermatitis. In stasis dermatitis barrier dysfunction is due to lower extremity edema.

Barrier dysfunction permits environmental microbes and chemicals to trigger an innate immune response producing 'danger signal' cytokines which increase the risk of

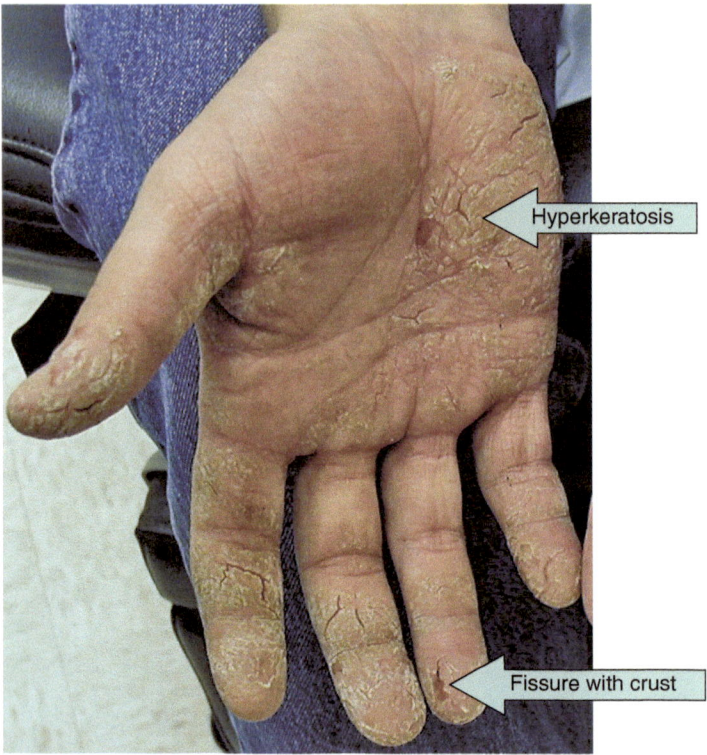

FIGURE 2.6 Chronic dermatitis

allergic sensitization [2]. Allergic contact dermatitis can then occur as a secondary cause of dermatitis in the atopic and/or irritant scenarios outlined in the previous paragraph (Fig. 2.7). In some cases, the sensitizer itself has irritant properties [3].

Allergic contact dermatitis to low-molecular weight antigens can be described as a type IV (delayed type, T cell mediated) reaction. Protein allergens like latex and food allergens may require IgE assistance for antigen presentation and this

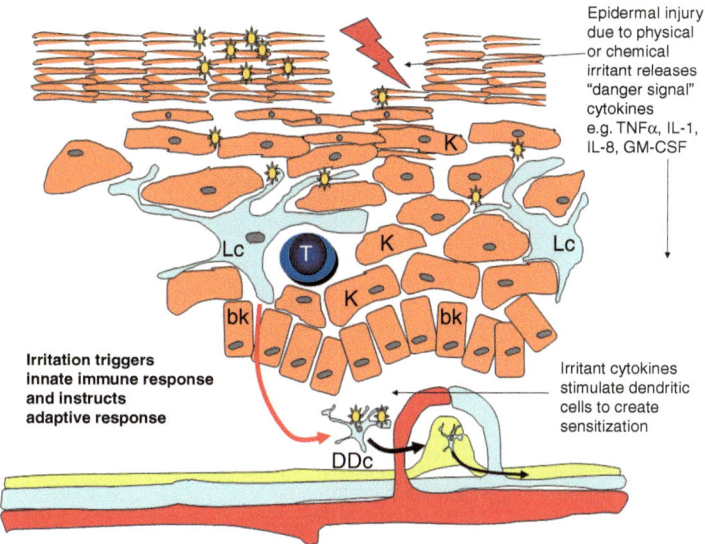

FIGURE 2.7 Irritation as danger signal. Key: *Lc* Langerhans cell, *DDc* dermal dendritic cell, *k* keratinocyte, *bk* basal keratinocyte

is described as mixed immune mechanism. These allergens are more common in atopic patients and often cause systemic contact dermatitis. Food allergy causing eczematous reactions is an example of systemic contact dermatitis as described in Chap. 4.

Diagnosis and Management

The cause of dermatitis is not revealed by the morphological appearance, although anatomic distribution can be helpful in determining cause. The history is the most important diagnostic tool for classifying dermatitis. Clinicians need to be able to discern sub-types of dermatitis from a context-rich history (Fig. 2.8). Management algorithms differ for subtypes

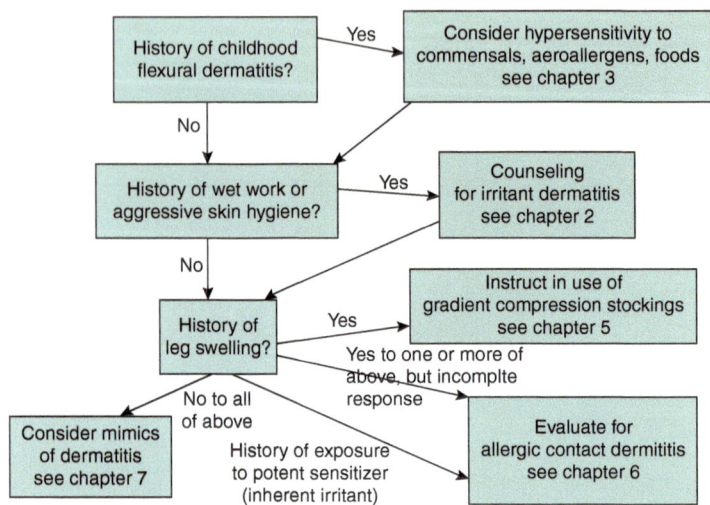

FIGURE 2.8 History guides diagnostic considerations

of dermatitis. Clinicians must be able to communicate deductive reasoning concerning diagnosis of dermatitis to patients, to colleagues, and in the medical record. Atopic dermatitis is most likely with a history of childhood flexural dermatitis. Adult onset atopic dermatitis is rare, and misdiagnosis can expose patients to the risks of immunosuppressive therapies when alternatives with less morbidity may be appropriate.

Although purely irritant dermatitis is common on the hands in workers doing wet work, generalized dermatitis is almost never purely irritant. Consistent exposures are usually the culprit for chronic irritant dermatitis which is often self-diagnosed by the patient.

Patients are familiar with irritant dermatitis because it is so common, and they assume that allergic dermatitis shares the features of requiring frequent and prolonged exposures. However, even short, occasional exposures can cause chronic allergic contact dermatitis. Patients must understand this before giving an exposure history.

Patient education must be provided at each stage of management to achieve best outcomes; this is especially important with evaluation of allergic contact dermatitis as most patients have a mental model of immediate type hypersensitivity and are unfamiliar with the concepts of delayed type hypersensitivity (Table 2.1).

TABLE 2.1 Patient education: evaluation of allergic contact dermatitis

Patient education before taking history	Rash appears days after skin contact, and can last for weeks even from a single, short exposure
	Contactants that feel soothing to the skin can be the source of allergy; and contactants that sting will not always cause rash
	You may be allergic to hypo-allergenic or "natural" products
	You may have more than one allergy, including allergies to items or medications used to protect or treat rash from an initial allergen
	You may have allergy to a substance transferred un-intentionally
Patient education before patch testing	Scratch testing detects allergens that are inhaled or ingested and cause immediate reactions; scratch testing cannot replace patch testing
	Skin takes days to produce an immune response; red spots indicating allergy may appear between 1 and 10 days after the patches are placed
	Patch tests remain on the skin for 48 h; marks indicating patch test placement must be kept dry until the test is complete (day 4–8)
Patient education after allergens identified	Rash will take approximately 4 weeks after last allergen exposure to improve 80%
	Complete avoidance of allergens is needed to see any improvement; partial avoidance will NOT result in partial improvement
	Treatment with corticosteroids will cause rash to temporarily disappear and make it difficult to interpret resolution from avoidance
	Ask your doctor about alternatives for products you cannot use due to allergy and whether protective equipment will be useful
	Dermatitis is often multi-factorial, and interventions in addition to allergen avoidance may be required to control your rash

Management of Itch

Patients often arrive for evaluation of generalized dermatitis frustrated and sleep-deprived. While undergoing diagnostic evaluation to determine the cause of their dermatitis, patients will often declare that they can tolerate the rash while undergoing more testing, but need relief for the symptom of itch. Table 2.2 lists educational points that may help to decrease patient frustration.

In patients with an urticarial/dermatographic component (usually patients with eczematous drug eruption, atopic dermatitis, or other systemic contact dermatitis) systemic anti-histamines are helpful. However, for most dermatitis patients, anti-histamines are useful only for sedative effect to improve sleep.

Systemic corticosteroids are helpful in most types of dermatitis, but interfere with diagnostic evaluation such as patch testing and quantification of peripheral eosinophilia. Topical

TABLE 2.2 Counseling generalized dermatitis patients about itch

Reassure the patient	Teach concepts
Frustration due to interference with sleep and concentration is normal	Stress worsens inflammatory skin disease and the skin disease increases stress
Adherence to all parts of the treatment plan can reduce symptoms of itch	There is no single cure for itch due to generalized dermatitis
There are few effective symptomatic treatments for itch	Itch, like pain, is worsened by stress. Itch is best controlled by treating the underlying disease
You will treat the itch after completing diagnostic evaluation	Treatments for itch can interfere with diagnostic testing
Immunosuppressive treatments will be used only when needed	Immunosuppressive treatments can be used in preparation for diagnostic testing, or rarely for long-term management (see Chap. 9)

corticosteroids rarely sufficiently control severe eczema and may cause secondary allergic contact sensitization. Neither systemic nor topical corticosteroids should be used as monotherapy long-term but are useful for short-term control of itch. Failure to respond to systemic corticosteroids is an important diagnostic clue as it is suggestive of mimics of dermatitis such as dermatitis herpetiformis (gluten sensitivity) or myelocytic hypereosinophilic syndrome.

Topical counter-irritants such as menthol and camphor, especially when chilled, are of limited benefit but do not complicate the diagnostic process.

Dermatitis and the Health Care System

Multi-factorial disease requires multiple concurrent treatments for flares and long-term use of simultaneous preventive maneuvers. Physicians and patients must attend to:

1. Barrier repair
2. Allergy
3. Infection

Comparative effectiveness studies are difficult because attention to only one of these factors with neglect of the other will obscure potential benefit. Real-world efficacy studies are needed, but very few exist.

Precise identification of patient cohorts that allows for co-existence of different subtypes of dermatitis can improve management and research of dermatitis (Fig. 2.9).

Appreciation of the subtypes and mechanisms of dermatitis will allow us to improve public health (e.g. better timing of introduction of solid foods for infants at risk of atopic dermatitis, better occupational hygiene, and reduction of sensitizers in personal care products and textiles). Awareness of the complexities of dermatitis may also encourage interdisciplinary collaboration between allergists, dermatologists, primary care physicians, nurses, dieticians, and psychologists resulting in better patient care (see Chap. 11).

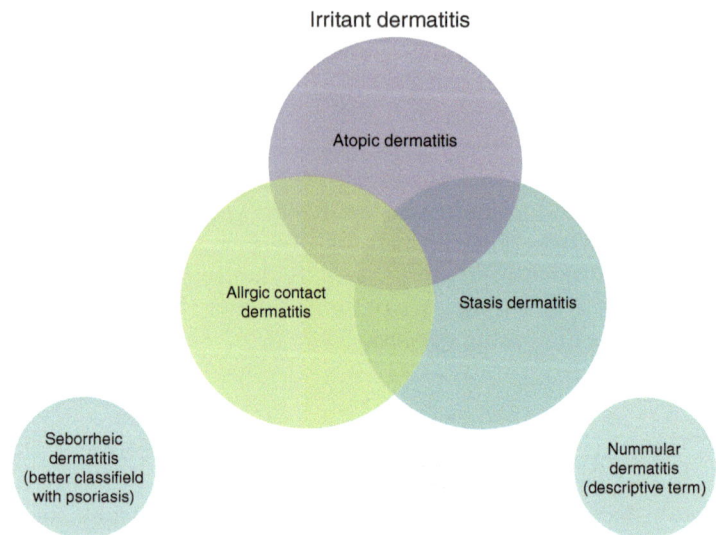

FIGURE 2.9 Irritant dermatitis underlies other types of dermatitis

References

1. Irvine AD, McLean WH, Leung DY. Filaggrin mutations associated with skin and allergic diseases. N Engl J Med. 2011;365(14):1315–27.
2. Matzinger P. Tolerance, danger, and the extended family. Annu Rev Immunol. 1994;12:991–1045 (Volume publication date April 1994).
3. Basketter DA, Kan-King-Yu D, Dierkes P, Jowsey IR. Does irritation potency contribute to the skin sensitization potency of contact allergens? Cutan Ocul Toxicol. 2007;26(4):279–86.

Chapter 3
The Role of Irritation in Dermatitis: Implications for Treatment

Key Concepts

- Barrier dysfunction leads to innate immune response that instructs adaptive response
- Emollients dampen innate immune response, possibly increasing risk of malignancy in normal skin
- Corticosteroids should not be used long-term to treat irritant dermatitis

Definition

Irritant dermatitis is the result of chemical or mechanical damage to keratinocytes with inflammatory response mediated by the innate immune response. The circumstances of activation of the innate immune response are one of several factors that instruct the adaptive immune response.

Irritation and Innate Immunity

Irritation is the precipitating event for localized dermatitis. Irritation can occur from wet-dry cycles or from chemical irritants or from stretch of the skin. Generalized dermatitis is almost never purely irritant in nature, but all forms of dermatitis start with cutaneous irritation.

S.T. Nedorost, *Generalized Dermatitis in Clinical Practice*,
DOI 10.1007/978-1-4471-2897-7_3,
© Springer-Verlag London 2012

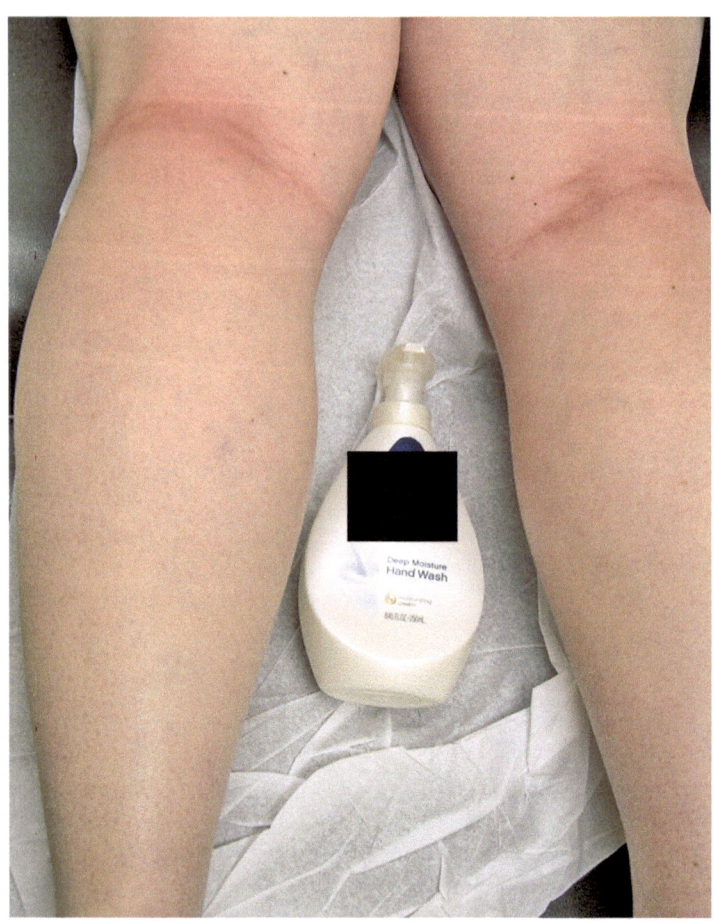

FIGURE 3.1 Acute irritant dermatitis accentuated in skin folds; the patient mistakingly applied a cleanser as a leave-on emollient

Pure irritant dermatitis is of mild to moderate severity clinically, and is accentuated in skin folds. Figure 3.1 shows acute irritant dermatitis from a body wash which the patient mistook for an emollient and left on overnight. This is an example of chemical irritant dermatitis. Patients often correctly diagnose irritant dermatitis themselves and may not seek medical attention.

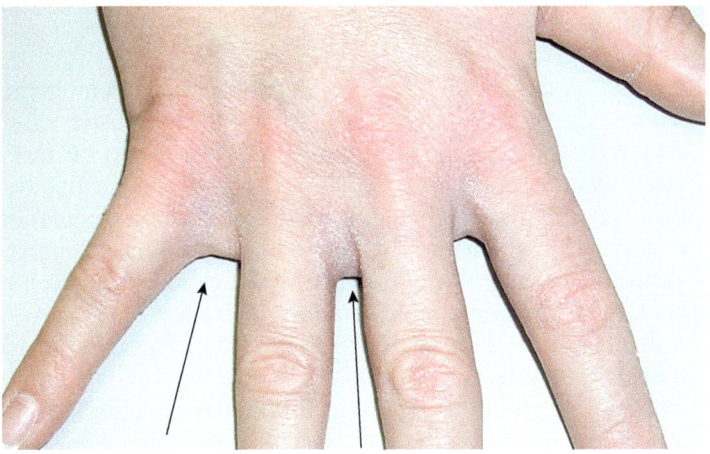

FIGURE 3.2 Chronic mild irritant dermatitis from prolonged use of occlusive gloves; occlusive gloves over cotton gloves are appropriate for wet work, but should be discourage for dry tasks in this postal worker

Figure 3.2 shows chronic interdigital irritation from prolonged maceration due to use of nitrile gloves during the winter by a postal worker. This is an example of irritation from wet-to-dry cycles which is more pronounced in low humidity environments when skin dries rapidly.

Because wet-to-dry cycles can cause epidermal damage, water is the most common irritant. Irritant dermatitis is also often due to excessive skin hygiene in areas of thin epidermis such as the eyelid or genitalia.

Epidermal irritation can come from physical trauma (e.g. fissuring from rapid wet-dry cycles or scratching) or from stretch of the epidermis (e.g. stasis dermatitis), infection, or from environmental chemicals. Many allergens are also irritants: dust mites contain proteases that decrease barrier function and are countered by endogenous protease inhibitors [1]. The innate immune system senses irritants and differentially instructs the adaptive immune system such that irritants have an effect on allergic response [2].

Emollients

Irritant dermatitis can be subdued by application of emollients that restore epidermal barrier function. More occlusive emollients such as ointments are generally believed to be more potent than less occlusive emollients such as lotions. In addition to restoring barrier function, occlusion blocks up-regulation of nerve growth factor that occurs after epidermal injury; occlusion does not block up-regulation of cytokines and can in fact induce inflammation in some circumstances [3].

Protection from rapid drying in low humidity conditions is critical. Patients are often advised to apply emollients immediately after bathing to 'lock in the moisture', although the importance of the timing is in fact to slow evaporation from the surface that can lead to fissuring in low humidity conditions. This is demonstrated by the exclusively seasonal occurrence of irritant hand dermatitis in health care workers in the Midwestern US in winter [4]. An analogy to mud cracking with rapid, but not with slow, drying is useful when educating patients. Use of alcohol-based hand sanitizers in low humidity conditions may decrease the incidence of irritant hand dermatitis by reducing the number of wet-to-dry cycles from handwashing [5].

Washing with soaps and disinfectants causes increased pH and enhances the activity of proteases and decreases the activity of lipid synthesis enzymes [6] leading to impaired barrier function. Alkalization due to washing may contribute to the localization of atopic dermatitis to skin folds. Acidifying the stratum corneum of dermatitis prone mice does not prevent oxazalone sensitization, but maintaining low pH decreases the intensity of dermatitis with prolonged antigen exposure, presumably because of improved barrier function [7]. Acidic emollients are preferred to pH neutral products, but are difficult for consumers to identify. They are often marketed as "pH balanced".

Emollients containing ceramides may most closely mimic the ceramide, cholesterol, and fatty acid lipid barrier of the intact stratum corneum [8]. They are more expensive than purely petrolatum based emollients and most are preserved with quaternary ammonium compounds. These preservatives are not routinely tested when screening for allergic contact dermatitis. It is therefore important to test to patient's own products in addition to a standard screening series.

Because of the risk of secondary allergic sensitization, emollients containing sensitizers such as fragrance should be avoided. Ointments may sting less upon application to inflamed skin than lotions, and require fewer potentially sensitizing preservatives because of the lower water content. However, very occlusive emollients can increase inflammation especially if deficits in innate immune function predispose to microbial proliferation under the occlusion.

Heavy emollients based on petrolatum require fewer preservatives but can create occlusion that may allow proliferation of commensal skin bacteria and yeast and may thus worsen dermatitis. This is of particular concern in atopic dermatitis patients who lack some anti-microbial peptides that predispose them to staphylococcal infections [9]. Many atopic patients complain of increased itch in humid weather with use of ointment-based topicals.

Finally, emollients should be used with caution in normal skin. The innate immune system is important for control of neoplasia. Emollients have been noted to increase number of skin tumors after UVB radiation in susceptible mice [10].

Textiles

Textiles are part of the cutaneous environment, and can influence immune response. Although occlusion is almost always useful in psoriasis where anti-microbial peptide function is normal, occlusion can be detrimental in dermatitis (Fig 3.3). "Sauna suits" made of occlusive vinyl were popular for psoriasis treatment in the 1980s, but should never be used for dermatitis patients.

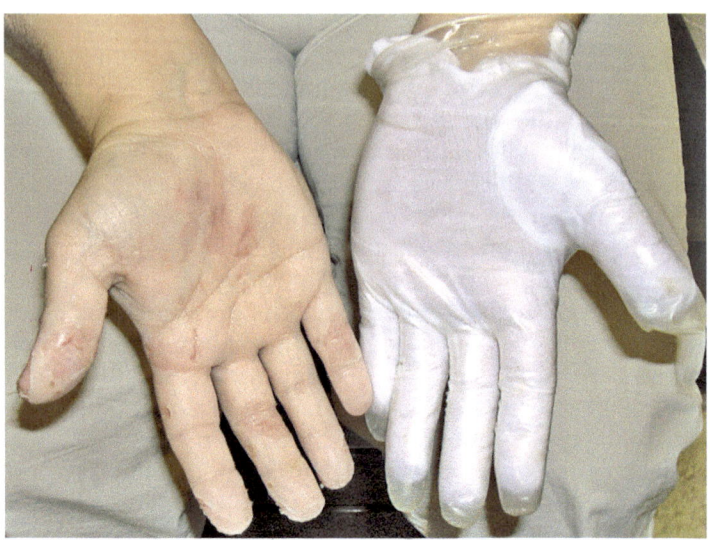

FIGURE 3.3 Irritant dermatitis atop dyshidrotic eczema in a patient who wore cotton OVER occlusive gloves, rather than under them to absorb perspiration

Textiles that wick moisture from the skin such as woven cotton or lyocell are better tolerated than occlusive textiles such as filament polyester. Textiles that contain anti-microbials such as nano-particles of silver can also be helpful for dermatitis patients, although long-term safety data is lacking for many items utilizing nano-technology.

Influence of Innate Immunity on the Adaptive Immune Response

Several variables influence the adaptive response. Mice with engineered deficits in the innate immune response cannot mount effective irritant or allergic contact dermatitis, demonstrating the importance of the innate immune system in instructing the adaptive response in allergic contact dermatitis [11].

Nature of the Allergen

The nature of the antigen is important. Many cutaneous allergens cause exclusively delayed type (T cell mediated) hypersensitivity. Some antigens such as toluene diisocyanate (TDI), can cause both dermatitis (usually considered delayed type allergy) and asthma (usually considered immediate type). See Chap. 6 for discussion of generalized allergic contact dermatitis in conjunction with asthma from two other such allergens—ammonium persulfate and potassium peroxymonosulfate.

Type of Tissue First Exposed and Concentration of Allergen

In the absence of co-stimulatory molecules, tolerance rather than sensitization develops. Mucosal epithelium lacks co-stimulatory molecules, so initial exposure to a potential allergen on mucosa will induce tolerance (critical to preventing food allergy and allowing survival of our species!), while exposure on inflamed skin will lead to sensitization.

Mice exposed to the aforementioned TDI on mucosa before skin exposure become tolerant. Mice initially exposed epicutaneously to low concentrations of TDI develop asthma with subsequent pulmonary exposure, while mice who received high concentrations on three subsequent days did not, although both dermal exposures led to dermal hypersensitivity [12]. Thus, the concentration of allergen at first exposure may also influence the subsequent immunological response in terms of Th1/Th2 balance.

Other Variables

The number of variables that influence the instruction of the adaptive immune response creates complexity. [13].

Cutaneous response to the same antigen at the same concentration and same tissue may differ based on pre-existing inflammation, ultraviolet light exposure, and psychogenic stress. This complexity hinders pharmacological attempts to treat dermatitis, as there are a number of permutations of immune response and not all target responses are present in all cases.

Corticosteroids

Corticosteroids are widely used to treat dermatitis as they are broadly immunosuppressive. However, systemic corticosteroids have many deleterious side effects such as osteopenia and weight gain. Topical corticosteroids thin the epidermis and may reduce the irritancy threshold; they were not helpful in an experimental model of sodium lauryl sulfate induced dermatitis in humans [14]. Topical corticosteroid application in mice can increase itch from irritants via production of substance P [15].

In some areas of skin such as the face and genitalia, withdrawal of chronic corticosteroid application in humans creates intense burning known as steroid addiction syndrome. Therefore, corticosteroids should not be used long-term to treat irritant dermatitis.

The Role of Irritant Dermatitis in Generalized Dermatitis

Generalized dermatitis is often systemic or 'endogenous'. The immune mechanism of broken tolerance that leads to systemic contact dermatitis is unknown. This is further discussed in Chap. 5. However, it is important when evaluating any dermatitis to address the contribution of irritation. Table 3.1 summarizes recommendations for skin care in dermatitis.

TABLE 3.1 Skin care for dermatitis

Do	Do not
Apply low pH (often marketed as "balanced") and ceramide containing emollients to inflamed skin	Extrapolate data from inflamed skin; it may not be beneficial to apply emollients to normal, sun-exposed skin
Apply emollients while skin is still damp	Apply emollients under occlusion or in humid weather
Use alcohol based hand sanitizers	Wash hands more often than necessary
Wear knit clothing with soft fibers that wick moisture	Wear shiny filament fibers that trap moisture, or rough wool fibers
Use anti-microbial powders or cotton fabrics under occlusive protective equipment	Wear occlusive protective equipment directly on the skin (e.g. gloves, soccer shin guards, etc.)
Apply corticosteroids for short durations in conjunction with other measures to control dermatitis	Apply corticosteroids long-term or as the only treatment for dermatitis
Use dedicated products to remove cosmetics from eyelids	Wash and apply emollients with eyes closed exposing eyelids to products not intended for use at sensitive sites

References

1. Takai T, Ikeda S. Barrier dysfunction caused by environmental proteases in the pathogenesis of allergic diseases. Allergol Int. 2011;60(1):25–35. Review.
2. Kono H, Rock KL. How dying cells alert the immune system to danger. Nat Rev Immunol. 2008;8(4):279–89. Epub 2008 Mar 14. Review.

3. Elias PM. Stratum corneum defensive functions: an integrated view. J Invest Dermatol. 2005;125(2):183–200.
4. Welsh A, Baron E, Fekedulegn D, Kashon M, Yucesoy B, Johnson VJ, Santo Domingo D, Kirkland B, Luster M, Nedorost S. Winter season, frequent handwashing, and increased sensitivity to irritation from detergents are independently associated with hand dermatitis in healthcare workers. Manuscript in submission.
5. Löffler H, Kampf G, Schmermund D, Maibach HI. How irritant is alcohol? Br J Dermatol. 2007;157(1):74–81.
6. Cork MJ, Danby SG, Vasilopoulos Y, Hadgraft J, Lane ME, Moustafa M, Guy RH, Macgowan AL, Tazi-Ahnini R, Ward SJ. Epidermal barrier dysfunction in atopic dermatitis. J Invest Dermatol. 2009;129(8):1892–908.
7. Hatano Y, Man MQ, Uchida Y, Crumrine D, Scharschmidt TC, Kim EG, Mauro TM, Feingold KR, Elias PM, Holleran WM. Maintenance of an acidic stratum corneum prevents emergence of murine atopic dermatitis. J Invest Dermatol. 2009;129(7):1824–35.
8. Elias PM. Skin barrier function. Curr Allergy Asthma Rep. 2008;8(4):299–305. Review.
9. Ong PY, Ohtake T, Brandt C, Strickland I, Boguniewicz M, Ganz T, Gallo RL, Leung DY. Endogenous antimicrobial peptides and skin infections in atopic dermatitis. N Engl J Med. 2002;347(15):1151–60.
10. Lu YP, Lou YR, Xie JG, Peng Q, Shih WJ, Lin Y, Conney AH. Tumorigenic effect of some commonly used moisturizing creams when applied topically to UVB-pretreated high-risk mice. J Invest Dermatol. 2009;129(2):468–75 (note several subsequent comments and author replies).
11. Zhang L, Tinkle SS. Chemical activation of innate and specific immunity in contact dermatitis. J Invest Dermatol. 2000; 115(2):168–76.
12. Vanoirbeek JA, Tarkowski M, Ceuppens JL, Verbeken EK, Nemery B, Hoet PH. Respiratory response to toluene diisocyanate depends on prior frequency and concentration of dermal sensitization in mice. Toxicol Sci. 2004;80(2):310–21.
13. Clark R, Kupper T. Old meets new: the interaction between innate and adaptive immunity. J Invest Dermatol. 2005; 125(4):629–37.
14. Levin C, Zhai H, Bashir S, Chew AL, Anigbogu A, Stern R, Maibach H. Efficacy of corticosteroids in acute experimental irritant contact dermatitis? Skin Res Technol. 2001;7(4):214–8.
15. Fujii Y, Sengoku T, Takakura S. Repeated topical application of glucocorticoids augments irritant chemical-triggered scratching in mice. Arch Dermatol Res. 2010;302(9):645–52.

Chapter 4
Atopic Dermatitis

Key Concepts

- Atopic dermatitis probably results from a mixed IgE and T cell response to protein allergens
- Commensal skin organisms create immune response in atopic patients
- Atopy patch tests may best diagnose contact dermatitis to proteins which can cause systemic contact dermatitis

Definition

Several sets of diagnostic criteria have been published (Hanifin and Rajka, The UK Working Party and Millennium Criteria) [1]. A history of childhood flexural dermatitis is the simplest diagnostic question in practice. Adult onset atopic dermatitis is very rare and is over-diagnosed. In the absence of a history of childhood flexural dermatitis, chronic pruritic dermatitis with asthma and/or positive atopy patch tests is suggestive of atopic dermatitis [2].

Sensitization to Food Protein Allergens

Severe atopic dermatitis and atopic dermatitis with asthma are associated in many populations with mutations in genes of the epidermal differentiation complex, especially filaggrin [3]. Impaired epidermal barrier predisposes to irritant dermatitis in areas with frequent wet dry cycles such as the perioral area of teething infants (Fig. 4.1).

S.T. Nedorost, *Generalized Dermatitis in Clinical Practice*,
DOI 10.1007/978-1-4471-2897-7_4,
© Springer-Verlag London 2012

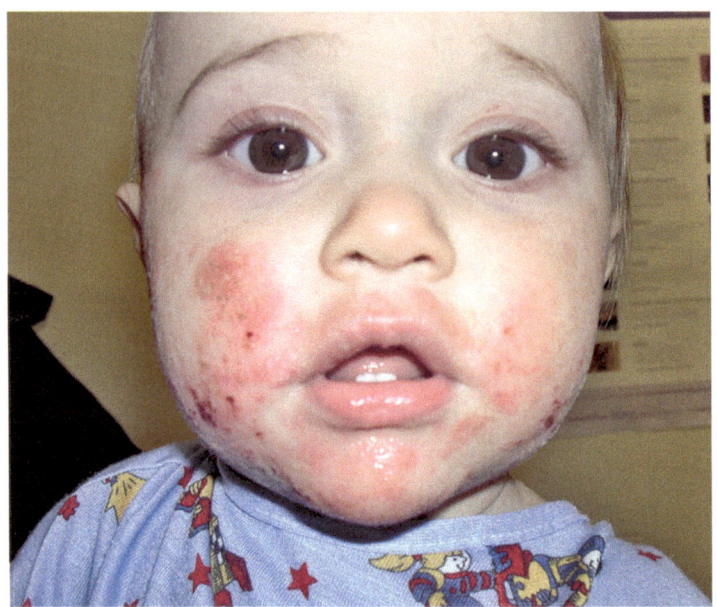

FIGURE 4.1 Perioral inflammation in an infant. Drooling provokes irritant dermatitis which increases risk for allergic sensitization

Impaired barrier function also allows for penetration of large molecules such as antigenic food proteins. If food proteins are first encountered on inflamed skin, rather than on mucosal surfaces with absent co-stimulatory molecules, then food allergy rather than tolerance may result [4, 5]. Filaggrin deficiency has been shown to increase the risk of peanut allergy [6].

The prevalence of peanut allergy is much lower in Israel at 0.06% than in the United States at 0.6%. In our inter-disciplinary eczema clinic (see Chap. 10), we speculate that this is due to ingestion of soft peanut snacks by Israeli infants that can be inserted into the mouth without skin contact. Peanut butter, on the other hand, is quite likely to stick to the perioral skin. In this sense, food allergy can be considered systemic contact allergy with sensitization via inflamed perioral skin (Fig. 4.2).

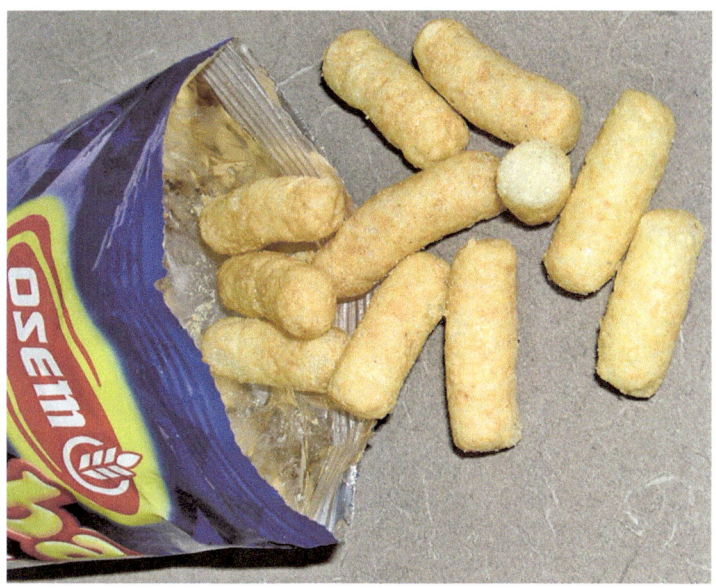

FIGURE 4.2 Soft peanut snacks that babies can dissolve in their mouths

In support of this model of food sensitization, a large German study showed no protective effect for atopic dermatitis or food sensitization (defined by tests for immediate hypersensitivity) of delayed introduction of solid foods beyond 4–6 months of age [7]. Subgroup analysis of children without infantile skin disease was carried out to exclude confounding changes in feeding behaviors due to diagnosis of atopic dermatitis, and this group had borderline significant protective effect of late introduction of solid foods. However, presumed lack of perioral inflammation in this group would be expected to dilute the protective effect of early mucosal exposure which is likely to be most important for children where perioral inflammation appears just prior to or coincident with the first exposures to solid foods. Although no studies have directly addressed this, it seems prudent to avoid introduction of new foods when perioral inflammation is present.

TABLE 4.1 Best practices as of 2012 to delay onset of atopic dermatitis and reduce food-triggered atopic dermatitis—not based on prospective data unless noted

Breast feed or feed highly hydrolyzed formula [8]
Introduce solid foods when child can digest them well
Attempt first food exposures directly onto the oral mucosa, discourage self-feeding new foods
Do NOT introduce new solid foods when perioral dermatitis is active
Introduce bananas, pitted fruits, potatoes, tomatoes before child begins outdoor play
Keep a pet dog indoors

Table 4.1 summarizes current best practices to reduce risk of food-triggered dermatitis in at- risk infants assuming that mucosal first exposure will promote tolerance and exposure on inflamed skin will promote allergy leading to dermatitis. Reduction of dermatitis due to foods may delay the 'atopic march' that leads to asthma and prolonged dermatitis.

Aeroallergens and after puberty, malassezia yeast, are later events that lead to further cross reactions and even autoimmunity to self-antigen. If the earlier food-triggered dermatitis can be avoided, there may be fewer danger signals from inflamed skin to promote the later events in the atopic march.

Sensitization to Pollen Protein Allergens

Keratinocytes can present allergens, especially in atopic patients and in the presence of inflammatory cytokines such as IL-4. Timothy grass pollen is taken up by keratinocytes in atopic skin [9]; inhalation of grass pollen triggering atopic dermatitis may then be another potential example of systemic contact dermatitis from cutaneous sensitization. Notably, atopic children develop flexural dermatitis at the same age when they begin to play outdoors (Fig. 4.3). Children with antigen-specific IgE to pollen report increased itch and extent of dermatitis during days with highest pollen counts [10].

Langerhans cells in atopic dermatitis patients with active disease bear Fc-receptor bound IgE, while Langherhans cells

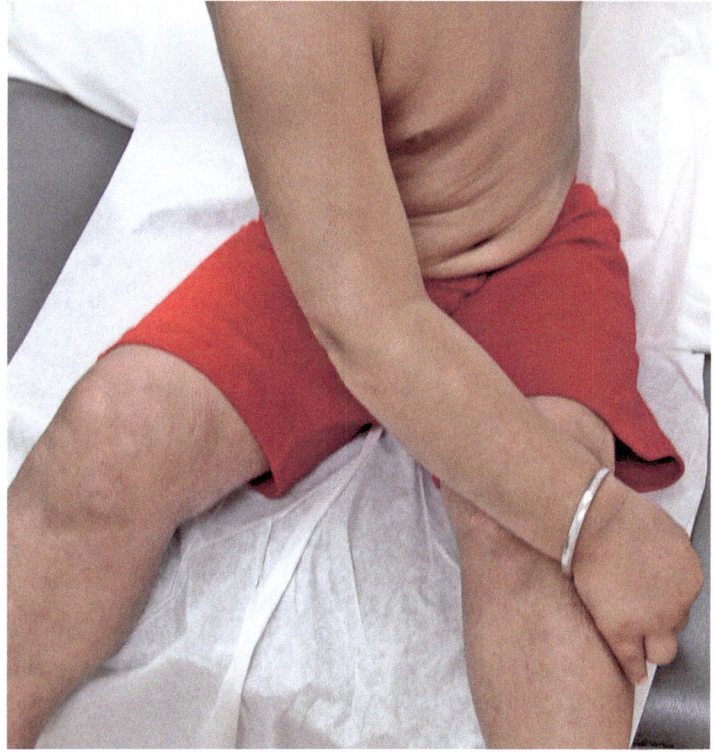

FIGURE 4.3 Child with positive patch test to compositae; note aeroallergen pattern

from normal non-atopic skin do not. These antigen-specific IgE molecules are important for aeroallergen presentation [11]. The type of T helper cell that is stimulated after antigen presentation likely depends on several factors including the nature of the antigen, type of antigen presenting cell, and type of antigen receptor. Figure 4.4 shows a simplified schematic of Th1 and Th2 responses.

Food Pollen Syndromes

Respiratory pollen sensitization can cause an IgE mediated tingling of the oral cavity when eating uncooked foods that share protein structure with the pollen; this is known as oral

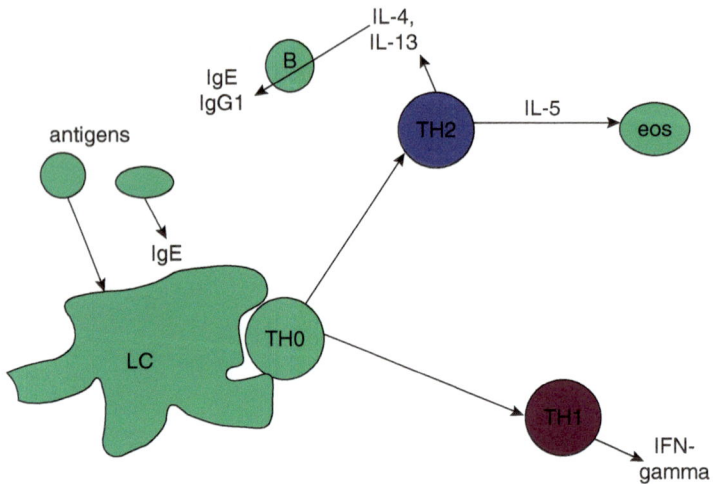

FIGURE 4.4 Th1 and Th2 differentiation

allergy syndrome. Latex sensitized patients have a similar reaction to foods such as kiwi [12]. However, T-cell mediated eczematous responses even to cooked foods can occur and are distinct from oral allergy syndrome. This is seen in older children and adults who have spring-time rhinitis and develop eczema after consuming birch related foods (Table 4.2) [13].

Cutaneous inflammation after antigenic ingestion or inhalation is called systemic contact dermatitis (see Chap. 7). T cells home to the tissue where the antigen was initially presented [14] T cells that home to skin express cutaneous lymphocyte antigen (CLA) and express the chemokine CCR4. CCL17 is a CCR4 ligand that is over-expressed in atopic dermatitis patients compared to healthy controls or psoriasis patients, suggesting a mechanism by which systemic antigen presentation may promote systemic contact dermatitis in atopic patients [15].

Atopic dermatitis patients who flare after foods related to birch pollen have a significantly higher number of CLA + lymphocytes after blood stimulation by birch pollen, but do not have higher levels of birch specific IgE compared to birch

TABLE 4.2 Frequency of food reactions (not limited to dermatitis) in patients with birch pollen allergy13

Food	Frequency of food hypersensitivity (%)[a]	Bet v 1 homolog
Apple	80.0	Mal d 1
Hazelnut	59.4	Cor a 1
Nectarine/peach	50.9	Pru p 1
Kiwi	47.9	Act d 8
Walnut	41.2	[b]
Carrot	34.5	Dau c 1
Apricot	33.3	Pru ar 1
Cherry	32.1	Pru av 1
Pear	32.1	Pyr c 1
Almond	31.5	[b]
Peanut	24.2	Ara h 8
Plum	24.2	Pru d 1
Tomato	21.2	[b]
Potato	18.8	[b]
Celery	15.8	Api g 1
Soybean	13.9	Gly m 4

Reprinted in part from Geroldinger-Simic et al. [13]. With permission of Elsevier
[a]Percentage of positive reactions in 225 patients with birch pollen allergy
[b]Not identified
Bet v 1 homologs and profilins in birch pollen–related foods

allergic atopic dermatitis patients who do not flare after ingestion of birch-related foods [16, 17].

Note that intact protein structures are required to stimulate B cells such that cooking allergenic foods will render them tolerable for many patients with immediate type food reactions. However, T cells that mediate delayed type allergy will recognize fragments of protein, such that even cooked foods may cause dermatitis.

Atopy Patch Tests: Concept

Atopy patch tests (APTs) predict delayed eczematous food reactions [18]. Many studies fail to differentiate early, non-eczematous reactions (gastrointestinal reactions, urticaria, etc.) from delayed, eczematous reactions; when these reactions are lumped together as 'food allergy', it is difficult to assess the diagnostic sensitivity and specificity of APTs. Lack of standardization of APTs has also contributed to controversy regarding their utility [19].

In a population exposed to oat in topical products, atopy patch tests frequently detected oat allergy in young children [20]. Stronger APTs (i.e. those with greater than 3 papules in addition to erythema and infiltration at the test site) predict food allergy even in teenagers and adults [21].

The lymphocytic and eosinophilic infiltrate in atopy patch tests is consistent with the histology of naturally occurring atopic dermatitis [22].

The NIAID-sponsored Expert Panel Report on Food Allergies published in 2010 made no recommendation regarding atopy patch testing for 'food allergy'; the panel did, however, recommend patch testing for systemic contact dermatitis [23]. Therefore, if atopic dermatitis is viewed as a form of systemic contact dermatitis to food and environmental proteins, atopy patch testing is currently the most practical diagnostic method for determining allergenic triggers of atopic dermatitis in that it assesses the ability of cutaneous dendritic cells and keratinocytes to present antigen. Although atopy patch testing is often used for patients with eosinophilic esophagitis, there are limitations in utilizing cutaneous antigen presenting cells as proxy for pulmonary or gastrointestinal antigen presentation, such that oral food challenge with observation intervals of at least 48 h to assess for delayed cutaneous reaction remains the seldom-used gold standard.

Atopy Patch Test: Procedure

Atopy patch tests are performed on non-inflamed skin of the back using 12 mm test chambers removed after 48 h [24]. Inspection of the test site should be delayed for at least

30–60 min after patch test removal; a 72 h inspection to assess for a crescendo pattern is helpful in equivocal reactions. As with conventional patch tests, there seems to be a correlation between strength of the reaction and specificity [25]. APT reactions with induration beyond the test chamber or more than 7 papules can be considered strong reactions. Figure 4.5 shows a strong reaction ragweed in the left column and a

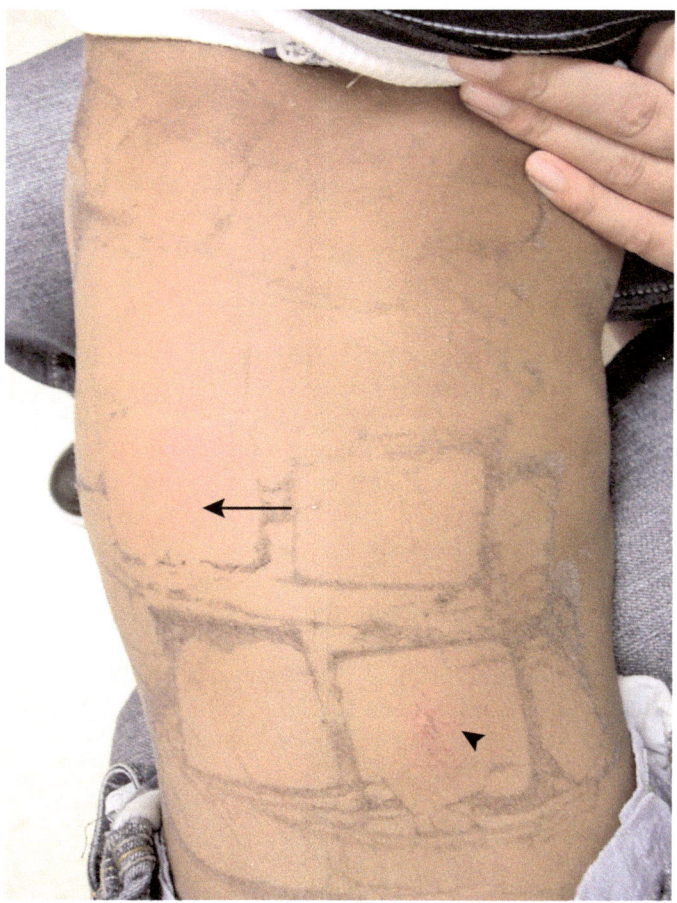

FIGURE 4.5 Ragweed reaction in left column, compositae reaction bottom right. *Arrow* is spreading infiltrated redness at raweed site. *Arrowhead* is weak reaction to compositae from coventional patch test series

cross-reaction to compositae mix at the bottom right site, and Fig. 4.3 shows the relevant clinical dermatitis in the same patient who experienced summertime flares.

Patients should not be tested to antigens until they have had exposure, both to prevent active sensitization and to reduce inhibition of oral tolerance [26]. In addition to restriction of systemic corticosteroids during the test interval and topical steroids and immunomodulators at the test site for 2 weeks before as in conventional patch testing, systemic antihistamines should be avoided during the testing interval. Table 4.3 compares atopy with conventional patch tests.

Atopy Patch Test: Patient Education

Avoidance of Topical and Ingestion Exposure to Foods

Atopy patch testing for food allergy is occasionally positive in adult atopic dermatitis patients who have never suspected food allergy (Fig. 4.6). There is very limited data on atopy patch testing in adults, but the technique may be underutilized. Food avoidance can be accomplished with expert dietary instruction, and data on the relevance of positive food atopy patch tests should emerge within the next few years.

Note that atopy patch testing to food is also relevant to food products used in personal care products such as oat and wheat proteins. Avoidance of hydrolyzed wheat protein in hair care products has been helpful to patients with facial and neck dermatitis and a positive atopy patch test to wheat.

Avoidance of Aeroallergens

Avoidance of aeroallergens in patients with positive atopy patch tests is more difficult. Figure 4.7 shows a positive atopy patch test to birch in a child who flared in spring and summer;

TABLE 4.3 Comparison of atopy and conventional patch tests

	Atopy patch test	Conventional patch test
Population tested	Suspected atopic dermatitis	Suspected allergic contact dermatitis +/− atopic dermatitis
Patch tests	Proteins formulated to desired PNUs by investigator; dust mite is commercially available	Commercially available; some FDA approved
Chamber size	12 mm	6 mm
Duration of patch contact with skin	48 h	48 h
Time to appearance of reaction	2–72 h	1–7 days
Morphology of reaction	Small papules, coalescent in strong reactions	Indurated erythema, vesicles, bullae in strong reactions
Possible mechanism	Keratinocyte or dendritic cell antigen presentation via IgE receptors stimulating T cell response	Dendritic cell presentation without assistance of IgE receptors stimulating T cell response

this child did not have oral allergy syndrome. Staying indoors with the windows closed and applying bentonite-based barrier cream marketed for poison ivy prophylaxis leads to anecdotal improvement in a number of such patients. Bentonite is derived from clay and adsorbs proteins. The vehicle of the barrier cream creates stinging upon application and is therefore not recommended for children with erosive dermatitis.

Dust mite avoidance is very problematic, and may best be accomplished by relocation to climates unfavorable to dust

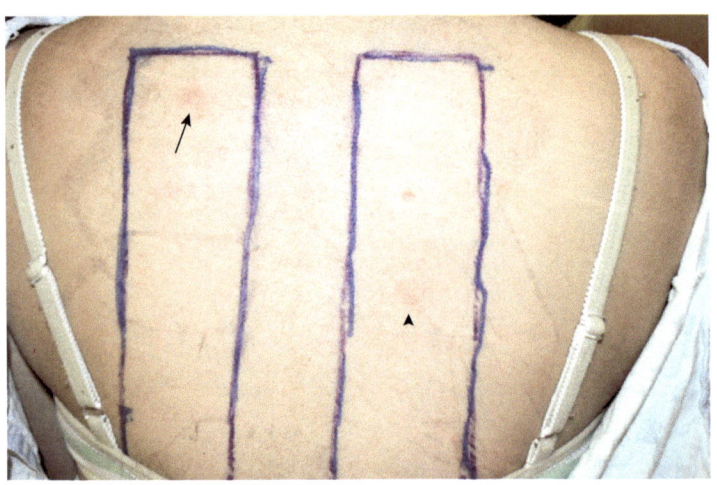

Figure 4.6 Positive APTs to cow's milk (*arrow*) and birch (*arrowhead*) in the setting of negative prick tests

mite, if feasible. However, this 'high altitude' therapy is better studied in respiratory atopy than in atopic dermatitis. There is data suggesting that at least for dust-mite triggered asthma and rhinitis, measures that only partially reduce dust mite exposure, such as impermeable bedding covers, are not beneficial [27]. Given the need for complete avoidance of cutaneous exposure of allergens to control allergic contact dermatitis, it seems unlikely that use of mattress and pillow covers alone to avoid dust mite is likely to make an impact on atopic dermatitis severity if upholstered furniture and carpeting remain in the home or are encountered outside the home. However, minimizing exposure to cutaneous irritants, which do not trigger an amplified adaptive immune response, is very helpful. To the extent that dust mites cause cutaneous inflammation by their protease activity, it may be useful to counsel atopic patients on avoidance.

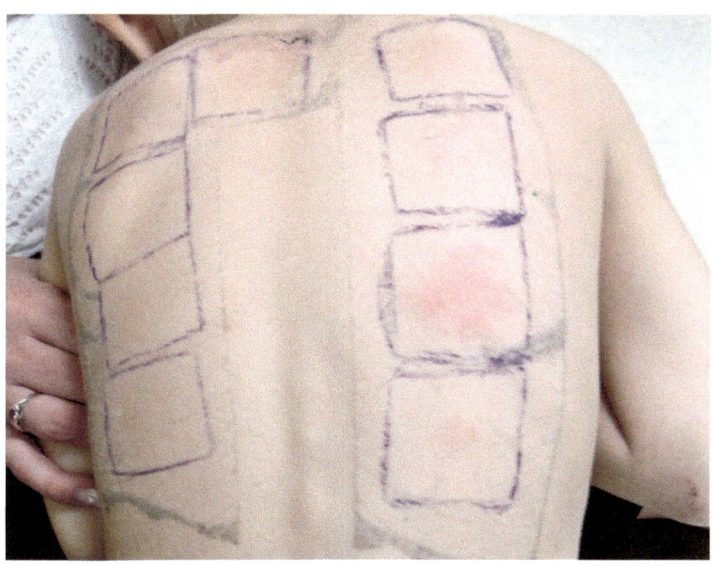

FIGURE 4.7 Positive atopy patch test to birch (second from *bottom right*) in child with springtime flares of atopic dermatitis (There is also a reaction of doubtful intensity to dust mite at the bottom right site)

Conventional Patch Testing in Atopic Dermatitis

Although atopic patients are harder to sensitize to non-protein allergens such as dinitrochlorobenzene under experimental conditions [28], they have large areas of chronically inflamed skin which is itself a risk factor for contact sensitization. Overall, atopic dermatitis patients have a very similar percentage of positive patch tests as non-atopic dermatitis patients, but they tend to have fewer reactions to potent sensitizers such as epoxy resin and neomycin, and more frequent reactions to compositae mix (possibly due to aeroallergen sensitization) and to tixocortal pivolate and propylene glycol (both components of many hydrocortisone creams and ointments) [29]. Dandelion (a member of the compositae family)

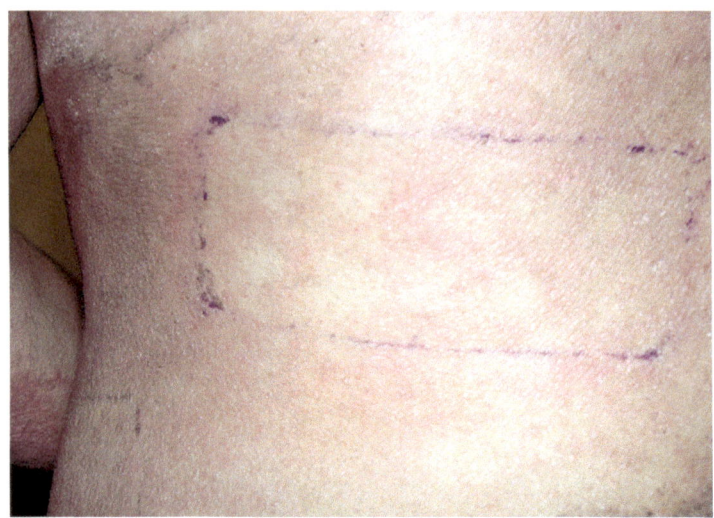

FIGURE 4.8 Flare of atopic dermatitis provoked by application of patch tests. There are no reactions within the test chambers which appear white

is a common sensitizer in young children [30]. Patients with positive patch tests to compositae or sesquiterpene lactone mix should avoid feverfew additives in "calming" emollients, although the manufacturers claim to attempt to eliminate allergenic components of feverfew.

Because occlusion can increase proliferation of commensal skin flora which may flare atopic dermatitis, systemic anti-yeast and anti-staphylococcal antibiotics may be useful before and during the patch test interval. Figure 4.8 shows a flare of atopic dermatitis provoked by patch testing.

Information on counseling patients with allergic contact dermatitis is provided in Chap. 6.

Role of Commensal Skin Flora in Atopic Dermatitis

Malassezia sympodialis yeast colonizes skin with sufficient sebaceous activity. In post-pubertal adults, these areas are the scalp, face, neck, and upper torso with accentuation at the anterior axillary line (Fig. 4.9). Atopic dermatitis patients can mount an immune response to these yeast confirmed by atopy patch test [31, 32]. There may be cross-reactivity between malassezia and human proteins recognizable by T cells [33]; this supports the concept that severe atopic dermatitis patients are reacting to 'self-antigen'.

Adult patients with atopic head and neck dermatitis show significant improvement with systemic itraconazole

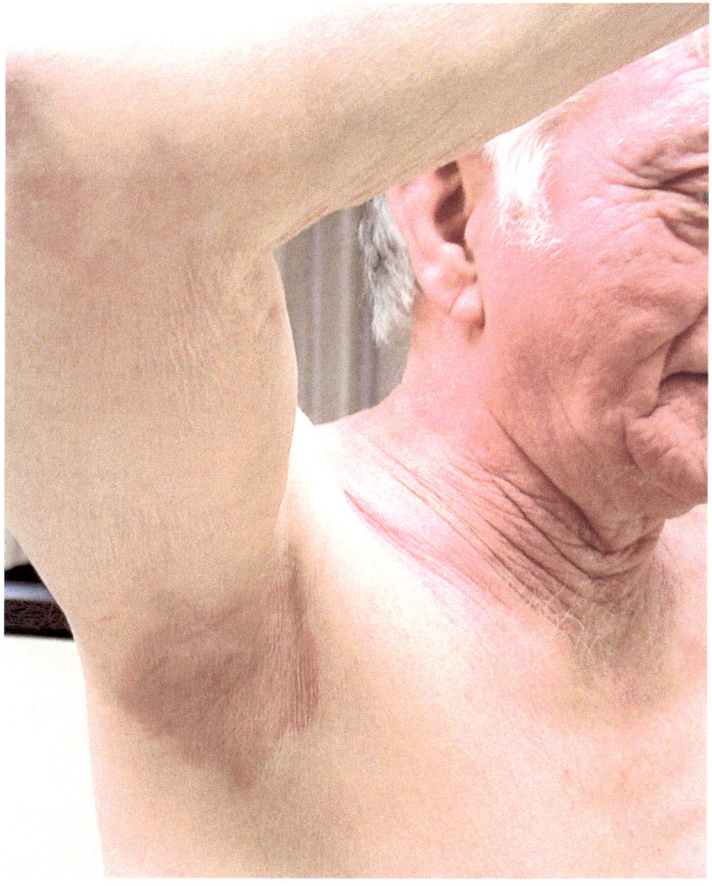

FIGURE 4.9 Adult atopic pattern dermatitis with head and neck and anterior axillary line involved

administered daily for 1 week [34]. In the clinical setting, routine use of ketaconazole shampoo to wash the upper body seems to lengthen the interval between required courses of systemic azoles to control head and neck flares.

Likewise, staphylococcus aureus worsens inflammation in atopic dermatitis patients. As discussed in Chap. 3, atopic dermatitis patients are deficient in antimicrobial peptides [35] and more than 90% are therefore colonized with staph. Staphylococcal bacteria initiate dendritic cell production of Th-2 chemokines and Th2 migration into the inflamed skin which further suppresses filaggrin expression and the ability of keratinocytes to mobilize the anti-microbial peptide beta-defensin, resulting in a cycle of increasing inflammation. In addition, staph endotoxins can function as superantigens and activate T cells and induce superantigen-specific IgE [36]. Anti-staphylococcal antibiotic treatment decreases inflammation in patients with atopic dermatitis [37]. Use of bleach baths after systemic antibiotics helps to reduce disease severity [38].

Staphylococci dominate the skin microbiome in the first few months of life and trigger immune responses considered normal such as erythema toxicum neonatorum; complex interplay between skin flora and the immune system may contribute to decreased prevalence of atopic dermatitis as children age [39]. This extends the prior knowledge that atopic dermatitis is more prevalent in urban than in rural areas (the hygiene hypothesis). In particular, exposure to farm animals and dogs, helminthic infections, and decreased exposure to antibiotics are all protective against atopic dermatitis [40]. Probiotics have been proposed as a preventive measure for high-risk infants, although a recent study of 3–6 month old infants with eczema at enrollment found to benefit of probiotic supplementation [41].

Table 4.4 summarizes clinical recommendations for care of young children with atopic dermatitis. Table 4.5 gives recommendations for management of teens and adults with atopic dermatitis.

TABLE 4.4 Management of young children with atopic dermatitis

Intervention	Rationale
10 days course of anti-staphylococcal antibiotics; based on culture and sensitivity	Decreases inflammation and will reduce the risk of flare with patch testing
Instruct in use of bleach baths	Slows re-colonization with staph
Use short course of systemic corticosteroids if child cannot tolerate baths and topical applications due to stinging	Adherence to treatment plan is poor if child has many erosions
Discontinue use of all current topicals except emollient free of common sensitizers	Topicals containing oat are associated with oat sensitization in many young atopic children
	There is no role for topical antifungals in young children with flexural dermatitis [42]
Apply antimicrobial powders to skin folds and under occlusive sports equipment such as shin guards	Occlusion worsens atopic dermatitis by encouraging proliferation of staphylococcus
Prescribe a structural group C topical corticosteroid without common sensitizers that has never been previously applied to the patient's skin:	Reduces risk of unrecognized allergic contact dermatitis to corticosteroids
Desoximetasone is a good choice; clocortolone cream is an alternative for patients who have used desoximetasone, although it contains rare sensitizers	
If child has a history of contact urticaria or anaphylactoid symptoms or respiratory atopy, perform skin prick or antigen-specific IgE tests	Testing for immediate hypersensitivity reactions should precede atopy patch testing to avoid test-induced anaphylaxis in high risk patients

(continued)

TABLE 4.4 (continued)

Intervention	Rationale
If child has a history of perioral eczema and has started to eat solid foods, perform atopy patch testing for foods	Atopy patch testing should be avoided in patients without risk factors as it may cause active sensitization or prevent induction of oral tolerance [26]
If child has begun outdoor play and has dermatitis on exposed skin, perform atopy patch testing to aeroallergen and sesquiterpene lactone or compositae mix and dandelion	Avoidance of food related to aeroallergens and use of bentonite based barrier creams may be useful in aeroallergen allergic patients
Mental health consultation for families who report significant impact of atopic dermatitis on quality of life	Habit reduction can reduce scratching behaviors; family counseling can be useful if family dynamics are affected by the attention the eczema demands

Wong et al. [42]; van Hoogstraten et al. [26]

Table 4.6 lists suggested atopy patch tests. In older children and adults, atopy patch testing is performed along with conventional testing to an extended screening series. In very young children, patch testing is difficult due to limited space on the back. Although it is always recommended to test an entire extended screening series, Table 4.6 also lists allergens that are most relevant in very young children at our center in the urban Midwestern United States. These allergens can be tested at the time of atopy patch testing for convenience if there is an appropriate exposure history. A delayed reading for the conventional patch tests is then needed in addition to the 'early' reading for atopy patch tests. Although fragrances are frequent causes of contact dermatitis, we do not attempt to screen for fragrance allergy in very young children as parents can readily find fragrance-free alternatives and have often instituted fragrance avoidance even before seeking medical attention.

TABLE 4.5 Management of atopic dermatitis in adult patients

Intervention	Rationale
10 day course of systemic anti-staphylococcal antibiotics based on culture and sensitivity	Almost all patients with active atopic dermatitis are colonized with staph
10 day course of systemic anti-yeast antibiotics for post-pubertal patients with head and neck dermatitis	Malassezia yeast requires oil for growth and thrives in sebaceous areas of skin after puberty
Instruct in regular use of bleach baths or swimming in a chlorinated pool. Rinse promptly after exiting pool or bath	Chlorine slows re-colonization of skin with commensals, but is an irritant
Wear clothing that wicks moisture; nanoparticle silver embedded in fabrics is useful for exercise wear; wash skin after perspiring	Occlusion worsens atopic dermatitis by encouraging proliferation of staph. and antigenic yeast
Prescribe topical corticosteroids from a structural class not previously used and without common sensitizers; use vehicle that patient prefers except avoid ointments in humid weather and avoid foams if propylene glycol allergy is suspected	Many adults prefer foam vehicles; these can be used on scalp and skin and do not stain clothing, but all contain propylene glycol. Many adults notice intolerance of occlusive ointment vehicles, especially in humid weather
Atopy patch test to food and aeroallergens unless contraindicated by history of immediate hypersensitivity (see Table 4.6)	Adults may have unrecognized delayed hypersensitivity e.g. to cow's milk or birch-related foods
Patch test to standard series and specific occupational series	Adults with atopic dermatitis have the same overall prevalence of contact allergies as non-atopic patients

TABLE 4.6 Suggested atopy patch tests for young children without suspected immediate type hypersensitivity

Suggested food atopy patch tests

Cow's milk

Soy

Wheat

Egg white

Oat

(Optional) corn meal

Suggested aeroallergen atopy patch tests

Bluegrass

Ragweed

Birch

Dust mite

(optional) dog, cat

Supplemental standard patch tests (if space precludes testing full series)

Sequiterpene lactone/compositae mix

Dandelion

(Optional) if corticosteroids previously prescribed: tixocortal pivolate; budesonide; propylene glycol; sorbitan sesquioleate

(Optional) quaternium-15; tocopherol acetate; cocamidopropylbetaine

References

1. Schram ME, Leeflang MM, DEN Ottolander JP, Spuls PI, Bos JD. Validation and refinement of the millennium criteria for atopic dermatitis. J Dermatol. 2011;38(9):850–8.
2. Samochocki Z, Owczarek W, Zabielski S. Can atopy patch tests with aeroallergens be an additional diagnostic criterion for atopic dermatitis? Eur J Dermatol. 2006;16(2):151–4.

3. Brown SJ, McLean WH. Eczema genetics: current state of knowledge and future goals. J Invest Dermatol. 2009;129(3):543–52.
4. Sabra A, Bellanti JA, Rais JM, Castro HJ, de Inocencio JM, Sabra S. IgE and non-IgE food allergy. Ann Allergy Asthma Immunol. 2003;90(6 Suppl 3):71–6.
5. Wennergren G. What if it is the other way around? Early introduction of peanut and fish seems to be better than avoidance. Acta Paediatr. 2009;98(7):1085–7.
6. Brown SJ, Asai Y, Cordell HJ, Campbell LE, Zhao Y, Liao H, Northstone K, Henderson J, Alizadehfar R, Ben-Shoshan M, Morgan K, Roberts G, Masthoff LJ, Pasmans SG, van den Akker PC, Wijmenga C, Hourihane JO, Palmer CN, Lack G, Clarke A, Hull PR, Irvine AD, McLean WH. Loss-of-function variants in the filaggrin gene are a significant risk factor for peanut allergy. J Allergy Clin Immunol. 2011;127(3):661–7.
7. Zutavern A, Brockow I, Schaaf B, von Berg A, Diez U, Borte M, Kraemer U, Herbarth O, Behrendt H, Wichmann HE, Heinrich J, LISA Study Group. Timing of solid food introduction in relation to eczema, asthma, allergic rhinitis, and food and inhalant sensitization at the age of 6 years: results from the prospective birth cohort study LISA. Pediatrics. 2008;121(1):e44–52.
8. Osborn DA, Sinn J. Formulas containing hydrolysed protein for prevention of allergy and food intolerance in infants. Cochrane Database Syst Rev. 2006;(4):CD003664. Review (cited in Table 1).
9. Blume C, Foerster S, Gilles S, Wolf-Meinhard B, Ring J, Behrendt H, Petersen A, Traidl-Hoffmann C. Human epithelial cells of the respiratory tract and the skin differentially internalize grass pollen allergens. J Invest Dermatol. 2009;129:1935–44.
10. Krämer U, Weidinger S, Darsow U, Möhrenschlager M, Ring J, Behrendt H. Seasonality in symptom severity influenced by temperature or grass pollen: results of a panel study in children with eczema. J Invest Dermatol. 2005;124(3):514–23.
11. Mudde GC, Van Reijsen FC, Boland GJ, de Gast GC, Bruijnzeel PL, Bruijnzeel-Koomen CA. Allergen presentation by epidermal Langerhans' cells from patients with atopic dermatitis is mediated by IgE. Immunology. 1990;69(3):335–41.
12. Kondo Y, Urisu A. Oral allergy syndrome. Allergol Int. 2009;58(4):485–91. Epub 2009 Oct 25. Review.
13. Geroldinger-Simic M, Zelniker T, Aberer W, Ebner C, Egger C, Greiderer A, Prem N, Lidholm J, Ballmer-Weber BK, Vieths S, Bohle B. Birch pollen-related food allergy: clinical aspects and

the role of allergen-specific IgE and IgG4 antibodies. J Allergy Clin Immunol. 2011;127(3):616–22.e1.

14. Clark R, Kupper T. Old meets new: the interaction between innate and adaptive immunity. J Invest Dermatol. 2005;125(4):629–37.

15. Esche C, Stellato C, Beck LA. Chemokines: key players in innate and adaptive immunity. J Invest Dermatol. 2005;125(4):615–28.

16. Reekers R, Busche M, Wittmann M, Kapp A, Werfel T. Birch pollen-related foods trigger atopic dermatitis in patients with specific cutaneous T-cell responses to birch pollen antigens. J Allergy Clin Immunol. 1999;104(2 Pt 1):466–72.

17. Werfel T, Reekers R, Busche M, Schmidt P, Constien A, Wittmann M, Kapp A. Association of birch pollen-related food-responsive atopic dermatitis with birch pollen allergen-specific T-cell reactions. Curr Probl Dermatol. 1999;28:18–28.

18. Kekki OM, Turjanmaa K, Isolauri E. Differences in skin-prick and patch-test reactivity are related to the heterogeneity of atopic eczema in infants. Allergy. 1997;52(7):755–9.

19. Lipozenci J, Wolf R. The diagnostic value of atopy patch testing and prick testing in atopic dermatitis: facts and controversies. Clin Dermatol. 2010;28(1):38–44. Review.

20. Boussault P, Léauté-Labrèze C, Saubusse E, Maurice-Tison S, Perromat M, Roul S, Sarrat A, Taïeb A, Boralevi F. Oat sensitization in children with atopic dermatitis: prevalence, risks and associated factors. Allergy. 2007;62(11):1251–6.

21. Celakovská J, Van cková J, Ettlerová K, Ettler K, Bukac J. The role of atopy patch test in diagnosis of food allergy in atopic eczema/dermatitis syndrom in patients over 14 years of age. Acta Medica (Hradec Kralove). 2010;53(2):101–8.

22. Bruijnzeel PL, Kuijper PH, Kapp A, Warringa RA, Betz S, Bruijnzeel-Koomen CA. The involvement of eosinophils in the patch test reaction to aeroallergens in atopic dermatitis: its relevance for the pathogenesis of atopic dermatitis. Clin Exp Allergy. 1993;23(2):97–109. Review.

23. Boyce JA, Assa'ad A, Burks AW, Jones SM, Sampson HA, Wood RA, Plaut M, Cooper SF, Fenton MJ, Arshad SH, Bahna SL, Beck LA, Byrd-Bredbenner C, Camargo Jr CA, Eichenfield L, Furuta GT, Hanifin JM, Jones C, Kraft M, Levy BD, Lieberman P, Luccioli S, McCall KM, Schneider LC, Simon RA, Simons FE, Teach SJ, Yawn BP, Schwaninger JM, NIAID-Sponsored Expert Panel. Guidelines for the diagnosis and management of food allergy in

the United States: summary of the NIAID-Sponsored Expert Panel Report. J Allergy Clin Immunol. 2010;126(6):1105–18.

24. Turjanmaa K, Darsow U, Niggemann B, Rancé F, Vanto T, Werfel T. EAACI/GA2LEN position paper: present status of the atopy patch test. Allergy. 2006;61(12):1377–84.

25. Heine RG, Verstege A, Mehl A, Staden U, Rolinck-Werninghaus C, Niggemann B. Proposal for a standardized interpretation of the atopy patch test in children with atopic dermatitis and suspected food allergy. Pediatr Allergy Immunol. 2006;17(3):213–7.

26. van Hoogstraten IM, von Blomberg BM, Boden D, Kraal G, Scheper RJ. Non-sensitizing epicutaneous skin tests prevent subsequent induction of immune tolerance. J Invest Dermatol. 1994;102(1):80–3 (cited in Table 4).

27. Terreehorst I, Hak E, Oosting AJ, Tempels-Pavlica Z, de Monchy JG, Bruijnzeel-Koomen CA, Aalberse RC, Gerth van Wijk R. Evaluation of impermeable covers for bedding in patients with allergic rhinitis. N Engl J Med. 2003;349(3):237–46.

28. Rees J, Friedmann PS, Matthews JN. Contact sensitivity to dinitrochlorobenzene is impaired in atopic subjects. Controversy revisited. Arch Dermatol. 1990;126(9):1173–5.

29. Nedorost ST, Babineau D. Patch testing in atopic dermatitis. Dermatitis. 2010;21(5):251–4.

30. Paulsen E, Otkjaer A, Andersen KE. Sesquiterpene lactone dermatitis in the young: is atopy a risk factor? Contact Dermatitis. 2008;59(1):1–6.

31. Johansson C, Sandström MH, Bartosik J, Särnhult T, Christiansen J, Zargari A, Bäck O, Wahlgren CF, Faergemann J, Scheynius A, Tengvall Linder M. Atopy patch test reactions to Malassezia allergens differentiate subgroups of atopic dermatitis patients. Br J Dermatol. 2003;148(3):479–88.

32. Ramirez de Knott HM, McCormick TS, Kalka K, Skandamis G, Ghannoum MA, Schluchter M, Cooper KD, Nedorost ST. Cutaneous hypersensitivity to Malassezia sympodialis and dust mite in adult atopic dermatitis with a textile pattern. Contact Dermatitis. 2006;54(2):92–9.

33. Balaji H, Heratizadeh A, Wichmann K, Niebuhr M, Crameri R, Scheynius A, Werfel T. Malassezia sympodialis thioredoxin-specific T cells are highly cross-reactive to human thioredoxin in atopic dermatitis. J Allergy Clin Immunol. 2011;128(1):92–99.e4.

34. Svejgaard E, Larsen PØ, Deleuran M, Ternowitz T, Roed-Petersen J, Nilsson J. Treatment of head and neck dermatitis

comparing itraconazole 200 mg and 400 mg daily for 1 week with placebo. J Eur Acad Dermatol Venereol. 2004;18(4):445–9.

35. Ong PY, Ohtake T, Brandt C, Strickland I, Boguniewicz M, Ganz T, Gallo RL, Leung DY. Endogenous antimicrobial peptides and skin infections in atopic dermatitis. N Engl J Med. 2002; 347(15):1151–60.

36. Ong PY, Leung DY. The infectious aspects of atopic dermatitis. Immunol Allergy Clin North Am. 2010;30(3):309–21. Epub 2010 Jul 1. Review.

37. Breuer K, HAussler S, Kapp A, Werfel T. *Staphylococcus aureus*: colonizing features and influence of an antibacterial treatment in adults with atopic dermatitis. Br J Dermatol. 2002;147(1):55–61.

38. Huang JT, Abrams M, Tlougan B, Rademaker A, Paller AS. Treatment of *Staphylococcus aureus* colonization in atopic dermatitis decreases disease severity. Pediatrics. 2009;123(5): e808–14.

39. Capone KA, Dowd SE, Stamatas GN, Nikolovski J. Diversity of the human skin microbiome early in life. J Invest Dermatol. 2011;131(10):2026–32.

40. Flohr C, Yeo L. Atopic dermatitis and the hygiene hypothesis revisited. Curr Probl Dermatol. 2011;41:1–34.

41. Gore C, Custovic A, Tannock GW, Munro K, Kerry G, Johnson K, Peterson C, Morris J, Chaloner C, Murray CS, Woodcock A. Treatment and secondary prevention effects of the probiotics *Lactobacillus paracasei* or *Bifidobacterium lactis* on early infant eczema: randomized controlled trial with follow-up until age 3 years. Clin Exp Allergy. 2012;42(1):112–22.

42. Wong AW, Hon EK, Zee B. Is topical antimycotic treatment useful as adjuvant therapy for flexural atopic dermatitis: randomized, double-blind, controlled trial using one side of the elbow or knee as a control. Int J Dermatol. 2008;47(2):187–91 (cited in Table 4).

Chapter 5
Stasis Dermatitis
and Autoeczematization

Key Concepts

- Barrier dysfunction from fluid pressure stretches skin and may expose self-antigen leading to autoeczematization.
- Patient education regarding the multi-factorial nature of dermatitis (barrier, infection, contact allergy) is even more challenging in this elderly and frail population.
- Compression or surgical intervention is necessary; topical medicaments alone are not sufficient.

Definition

Swelling of the lower leg stretches the skin and creates barrier disruption. As in other forms of dermatitis, innate immune response to barrier disruption then predisposes to allergic contact dermatitis. The increased vasculature and slow circulation in stasis dermatitis no doubt contribute to contact allergy, as the conditions required to break tolerance exceed the presence of danger signals alone [1].

Autoeczematization is defined as extension of dermatitis from the source site without explanation and often complicates stasis dermatitis.

S.T. Nedorost, *Generalized Dermatitis in Clinical Practice,* 53
DOI 10.1007/978-1-4471-2897-7_5,
© Springer-Verlag London 2012

Management of Stasis Dermatitis

Treatment of underlying causes that lead to leg swelling is important. Leg swelling may be multi-factorial and causes include: congestive heart failure, hypoalbuminemia, venous disease, and pharmacological side effects. Medications that contribute to leg swelling should be discontinued if possible. Amlodipine commonly causes lower extremity edema which is not alleviated by diuretics, but may be ameliorated by ACE inhibitors [2].

Misdiagnosis of cellulitis with unnecessary hospitalization and antibiotic treatment is common [3]. Bilateral leg involvement, lack of fever, and lack of leukocytosis are findings that argue against cellulitis. Bacterial colonization of the non-intact skin is common, and there is the risk of true infection from staphylococcus, pseudomonas, and other organisms. As in other forms of dermatitis, acute edema can produce bullae, which can also mimic blistering diseases.

Compression stockings are an inexpensive intervention with a good side effect profile, but compliance is poor [4]. Many patients need assistance to don the stockings. Mechanical assistive devices help a few, but often patients who live alone require a home health provider to be present when the patient arises. Stockings must be donned immediately after arising, before swelling can occur. Patients need to wear stockings whenever they are not in bed, even if sitting or sleeping in a recliner with legs partially elevated.

Venous surgery is increasingly utilized to improve venous stasis disease. This includes venous stenting [5] and ambulatory phlebectomy [6].

Secondary Allergic Contact Dermatitis

Allergic contact dermatitis is very common in the setting of stasis dermatitis [7]. In addition to the innate immune response to stretch in an area of skin without much laxity, gravity contributes to stasis that may slow blood flow and lengthens the amount of time immune cells spend in the cutaneous vasculature. The most common relevant allergens in patients with leg dermatitis in our center in the urban Midwestern United States are bacitracin/neomycin, fragrance mix, quaternium-15, Amercol 101/lanolin, and tixocortal pivolate as a marker for group A corticosteroids, but a number of other allergens are important as well including cetylstearyl alcohol, benzyl alcohol, and cocamide DEA. Figure 5.1 shows a patient with contact allergy to neomycin and bacitracin in triple antibiotic ointment referred for possible cellulitis.

Occasionally, patients will react to weak sensitizers such as paraben or lanolin when applied to inflamed skin on the lower leg, but not when applied on intact skin. This paradox can also result in false negative patch tests on intact skin [8].

Contact dermatitis to wound dressings can also occur. Modified colophony in hydrocolloids is a reported allergen, but patch testing to colophony on the standard series may be falsely negative either because of lack of cross reaction or because of the paradox of tolerance on intact skin [9].

Bland ointments that do not contain sensitizing preservatives, fragrances, or propylene glycol should be used for stasis dermatitis. If the patient requires a topical corticosteroid, a different structural class from previous usage should be selected to minimize the chance of allergic contact dermatitis [10]. Table 5.1 summarizes management of stasis dermatitis.

Autoeczematization

Patients with stasis dermatitis sometimes develop rapid extension of rash from the legs to the torso and upper extremities; since the 1920s, this has been speculated to be due to autoantibodies directed against skin [11]. In a mouse model, contact sensitization, but not cutaneous irritant exposure, generates T cells that react to keratinocyte antigen as well as to hapten [12]. Autoeczematization is observed in stasis

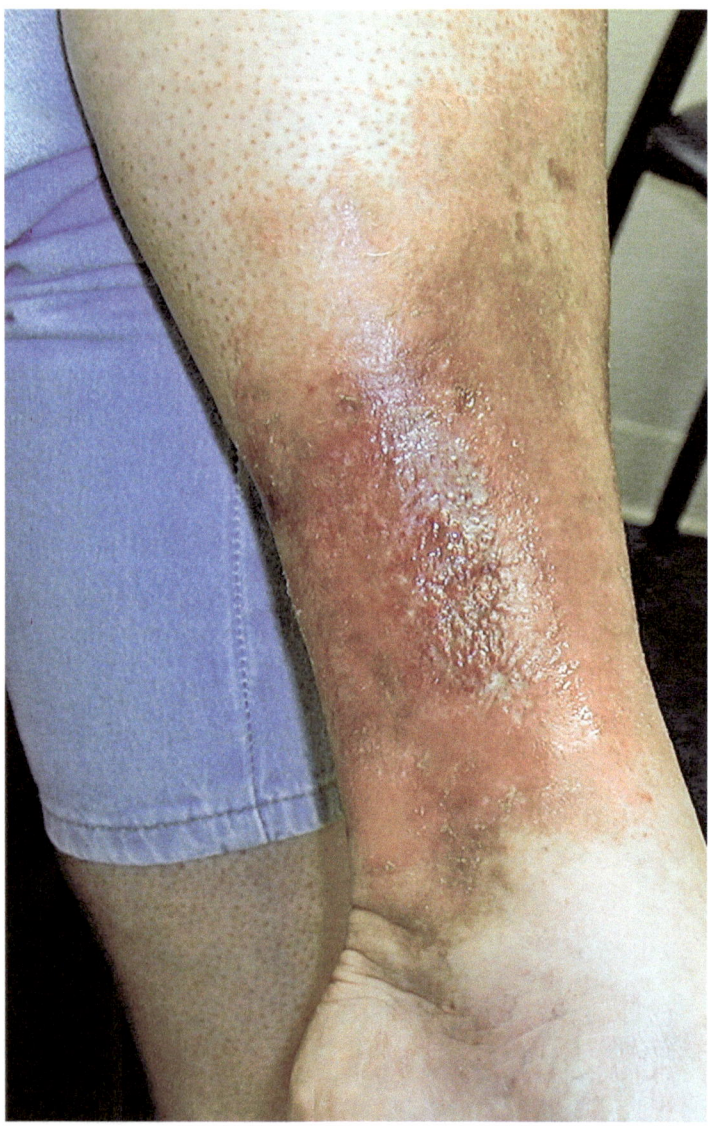

FIGURE 5.1 Allergic contact dermatitis due to neomycin and bacitracin thought to represent cellulitis by the referring physician

TABLE 5.1   Management of Stasis Dermatitis

Do	Do not
Optimize diet to normalize albumin, reduce fluid retention, and decrease obesity	Use diuretics as the only systemic intervention for lower leg edema
Arrange assistance to don compression stockings or apply paste boots	Utilize leg elevation as mainstay of treatment
Apply bland emollients such as petrolatum and non-sensitizing anti-microbials such as dilute bleach compresses	Apply emollients or cleansers with numerous ingredients
Prescribe halogenated, C16-methyl substituted corticosteroids when needed e.g. mometasone, fluticasone, betamethasone valerate, desoximetasone, dexamethsone [10]	Use structural associations of corticosteroids to replace patch testing of individual steroids in allergic patients
Consult for surgical intervention	Allow stasis dermatitis to progress to autoeczematization

dermatitis and in atopic dermatitis and allergic contact dermatitis in the form of excited skin syndrome that complicates patch testing. Systemic immunosuppressive treatment is often needed to suppress autoeczematization, and the condition often remits after such treatment.

Bullous Pemphigoid: An Instructive Mimic

Bullous pemphigoid can present as classic blisters or as an urticarial and eczematous disorder. The latter form is common, but difficult to diagnose as the specificity of immunoflourescent studies is less clear in these atypical variants [13]. This sub-bullous presentation often waxes and wanes with intermittent remissions but gradual progression over months. Short-term studies of treatment efficacy may be influenced by this unpredictable natural history.

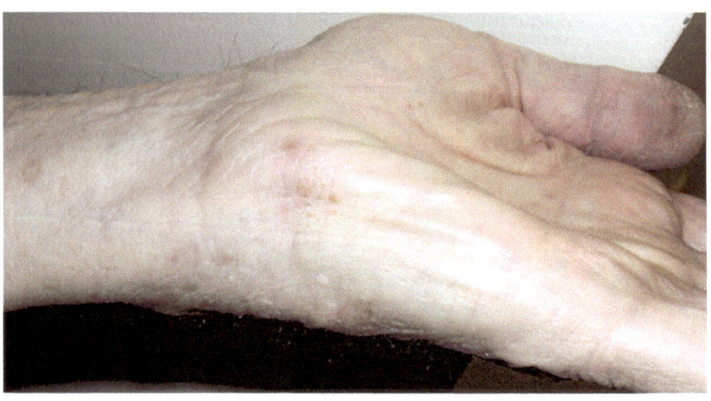

FIGURE 5.2 Linear IgA dermatosis with initial presentation on the palm mimicking dyshidrotic eczema

Both B and T lymphocytes target self-antigen; in early disease, epitope spreading, the development of antibodies to additional antigens, is common and correlates with severity of disease [14]. In some respects, bullous pemphigoid behaves as an autoeczematous progression with targeting of the basement membrane zone rather than the upper epidermal keratinocytes.

IgE antibodies to the basement membrane zone have recently been shown to have a functional role in the early phases of bullous pemphigoid independent of the IgE receptor [15]. There is also evidence for an IgE mechanism involving the high affinity receptor on mast cells and basophils given that the IgE receptor inhibitor omalizumab has been shown to reduce inflammation in a bullous pemphigoid patient [16].

There is sometimes great clinical similarity between dyshidrotic eczema and autoimmune bullous disease on the hands, which might also reflect the importance of IgE and other antibodies in autoimmune disease. Figure 5.2 shows a dyshidrosiform presentation of linear IgA dermatosis that illustrates the difficulty in distinguishing early bullous disorders from endogenous forms of dermatitis.

References

1. Holcmann M, Stoitzner P, Drobits B, Luehrs P, Stingl G, Romani N, Maurer D, Sibilia M. Skin inflammation is not sufficient to break tolerance induced against a novel antigen. J Immunol. 2009; 183(2):1133–43.
2. Gosnell AL, Nedorost ST. Stasis dermatitis as a complication of amlodipine therapy. J Drugs Dermatol. 2009;8(2):135–7.
3. David CV, Chira S, Eells SJ, Ladrigan M, Papier A, Miller LG, Craft N. Diagnostic accuracy in patients admitted to hospitals with cellulitis. Dermatol Online J. 2011;17(3):1.
4. Raju S, Hollis K, Neglen P. Use of compression stockings in chronic venous disease: patient compliance and efficacy. Ann Vasc Surg. 2007;21(6):790–5.
5. Alhalbouni S, Hingorani A, Shiferson A, Gopal K, Jung D, Novak D, Marks N, Ascher E. Iliac-femoral venous stenting for lower extremity venous stasis symptoms. Ann Vasc Surg. 2012;26(2):185–9.
6. Kundu S, Grassi CJ, Khilnani NM, Fanelli F, Kalva SP, Khan AA, McGraw JK, Maynar M, Millward SF, Owens CA, Stokes LS, Wallace MJ, Zuckerman DA, Cardella JF, Min RJ. Cardiovascular Interventional Radiological Society of Europe, American College of Phlebology, and Society of Interventional Radiology Standards of Practice Committees. Multi-disciplinary quality improvement guidelines for the treatment of lower extremity superficial venous insufficiency with ambulatory phlebectomy from the Society of Interventional Radiology, Cardiovascular Interventional Radiological Society of Europe, American College of Phlebology and Canadian Interventional Radiology Association. J Vasc Interv Radiol. 2010;21(1):1–13.
7. Machet L, Couhé C, Perrinaud A, Hoarau C, Lorette G, Vaillant L. A high prevalence of sensitization still persists in leg ulcer patients: a retrospective series of 106 patients tested between 2001 and 2002 and a meta-analysis of 1975–2003 data. Br J Dermatol. 2004;150(5):929–35.
8. Wolf R. The lanolin paradox. Dermatology. 1996;192(3):198–202. Review.
9. Goossens A, Cleenewerck MB. New wound dressings: classification, tolerance. Eur J Dermatol. 2010;20(1):24–6.
10. Baeck M, Goossens A. Immediate and delayed allergic hyper-sensitivity to corticosteroids: practical guidelines. Contact Dermatitis. 2012;66(1):38–45.

11. Cunningham MJ, Zone JJ, Petersen MJ, Green JA. Circulating activated (DR-positive) T lymphocytes in a patient with autoeczematization. J Am Acad Dermatol. 1986;14(6):1039–41.
12. Fehr BS, Takashima A, Bergstresser PR, Cruz Jr PD. T cells reactive to keratinocyte antigens are generated during induction of contact hypersensitivity in mice. A model for autoeczematization in humans? Am J Contact Dermat. 2000;11(3): 145–54.
13. Lipsker D, Borradori L. 'Bullous' pemphigoid: what are you? Urgent need of definitions and diagnostic criteria. Dermatology. 2010;221(2):131–4.
14. Di Zenzo G, Thoma-Uszynski S, Calabresi V, Fontao L, Hofmann SC, Lacour JP, Sera F, Bruckner-Tuderman L, Zambruno G, Borradori L, Hertl M. Demonstration of epitope-spreading phenomena in bullous pemphigoid: results of a prospective multicenter study. J Invest Dermatol. 2011;131(11):2271–80.
15. Messingham KN, Srikantha R, DeGueme AM, Fairley JA. FcR-independent effects of IgE and IgG autoantibodies in bullous pemphigoid. J Immunol. 2011;187(1):553–60.
16. Fairley JA, Baum CL, Brandt DS, Messingham KA. Pathogenicity of IgE in autoimmunity: successful treatment of bullous pemphigoid with omalizumab. J Allergy Clin Immunol. 2009;123(3): 704–5.

Chapter 6
Generalized Allergic Contact Dermatitis

Key Concepts

- Positive patch tests require assessment of relevance and knowledge of alternatives
- Negative patch tests require logical analysis and re-consideration of differential diagnosis
- Scabies is generalized protein contact dermatitis

Definition

Allergic contact dermatitis most often occurs in localized distributions such as the hands and face. Generalized allergic contact dermatitis denotes involvement of widespread areas such as the torso and extremities. Recognizable patterns such as photo-distribution or textile pattern suggest allergic contact dermatitis, but allergic contact dermatitis may also cause generalized dermatitis without a recognizable pattern.

S.T. Nedorost, *Generalized Dermatitis in Clinical Practice,*
DOI 10.1007/978-1-4471-2897-7_6,
© Springer-Verlag London 2012

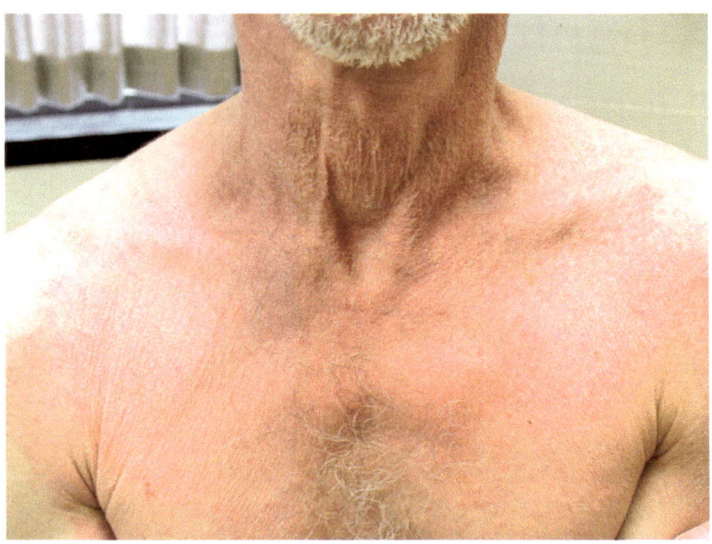

FIGURE 6.1 Machinist with dermatitis on hands as well as face, neck, and torso. He was sensitized to biocides and propylene glycol present in his metal-working fluids and personal care products

Causes of Generalized Allergic Contact Dermatitis

Sensitization to a Common Allergen(s) with More Than One Source, or Polysensitization

Patients allergic to formaldehyde releasing preservatives may react to several different personal care products and/or occupational sources, resulting in generalized allergic contact dermatitis. Figure 6.1 shows a machinist sensitized to a form-aldehyde- releasing biocide relevant to his metal-working fluids, propylene glycol relevant to his hand cleanser at work, and rubber accelerators relevant to his protective equipment. He also had contact allergies to corticosteroids

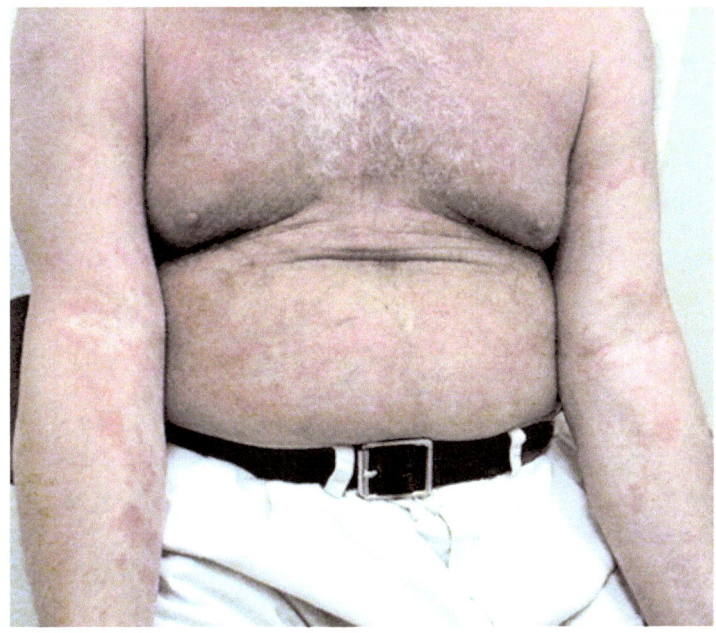

FIGURE 6.2 Generalized dermatitis from the neck down associated with recent onset asthma in a patient sensitized to potassium peroxymonosulfate in his hot tub

and antibiotics ointments. He had extensive involvement of his face, neck, torso, extremities, and hands at the time of patch testing.

Sensitization to an Allergen with Widespread Skin Contact

Figure 6.2 shows a patient sensitized to potassium peroxymonosulfate in his hot tub additive. He presented with generalized dermatitis sparing only the area above his neck and adult onset asthma, both of which resolved with avoidance of his sensitizer [1].

Contact Allergy as a Secondary Diagnosis Along with Other Dermatitis Such as Stasis Dermatitis with Autoeczematization or an Underlying Non-eczematous Skin Disease Such as Psoriasis

Spongiotic changes can obscure diagnostic pathology both clinically and histologically such that is sometimes impossible to diagnosis an underlying dermatosis until after contact dermatitis is controlled. Figure 6.3a, b show a patient with psoriasis and secondary allergic contact dermatitis.

Contact Allergy with Urticarial and Eczematous Response to Airborne Exposure

Figure 6.4a, b show a hairdresser with type 1 (wheezing and urticaria) and type 4 (positive patch test and dermatitis) hypersensitivity to ammonium persulfate used to bleach hair at her salon.

Patch Testing for Allergic Contact Dermatitis

There are excellent textbooks devoted to allergic contact dermatitis and patch testing [2–4]. Only general principles will be discussed here. Patch test selection varies by patient exposure. Even standard screening series must evolve over time as formulation of personal care products, textile finishing, and composition of popular medicaments change. Table 6.1 provides practical tips for patch testing.

Successful patch testing is dependent upon accurate pre-test suspicion for allergic contact dermatitis, appropriate selection of allergens based on the patient history, technical skill in applying and interpreting tests, ability to assess relevance of positive patch tests, and patient education resources for identifying alternatives to identified allergens,

Patch testing is the gold standard for diagnosis of allergic contact dermatitis. The most common reason for failure of patch testing to diagnose contact dermatitis is limitation of the number of allergens tested. Especially for occupational

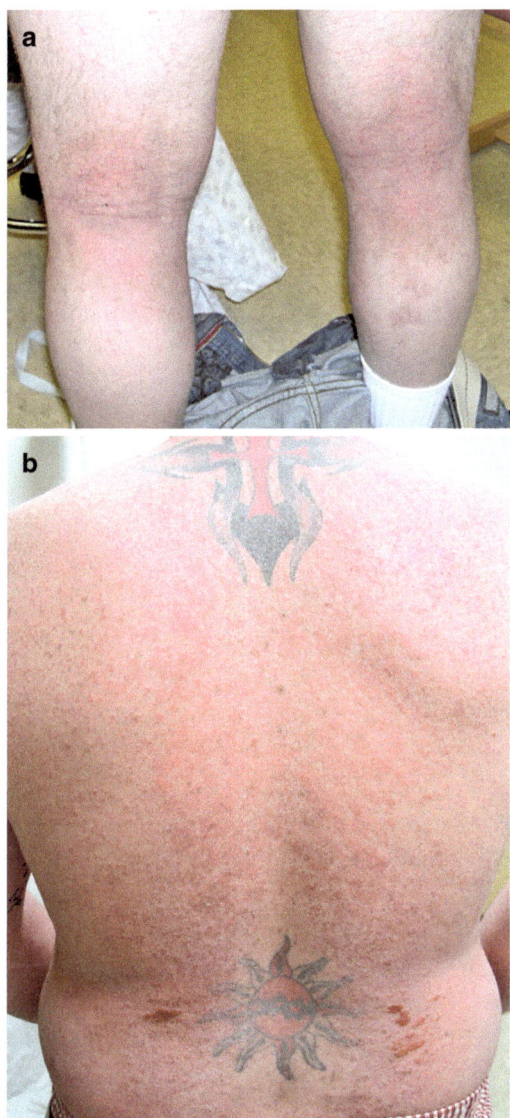

FIGURE 6.3 Psoriasis with widespread secondary allergic contact dermatitis. (**a**) Contact allergy masks psoriatic pattern. (**b**) This patient had contact allergy to aeroallergens and medicaments resulting in a generalized dermatitis atop his psoriasis

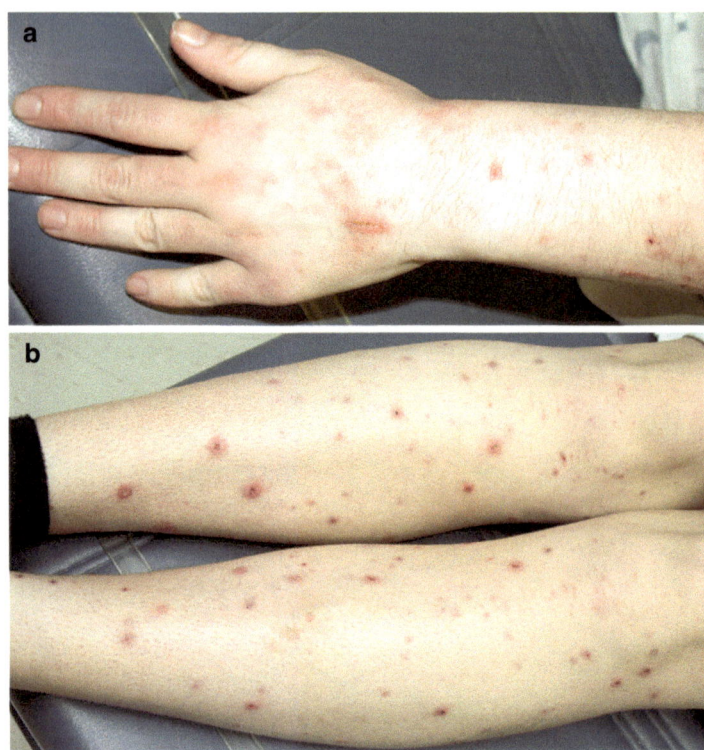

FIGURE 6.4 (**a**, **b**) Hairdresser with resolving generalized urticaria and hand dermatitis due to ammonium persulfate used to bleach hair at her salon. She needed to avoid both skin and airborne exposure

dermatitis, testing supplemental allergens beyond those considered standard allergens is essential. Limitations that may prevent adequate allergen selection include expense associated with stocking allergens that may expire before they are needed, expense in preparing allergens for testing, and lack of FDA approval for many allergens.

The most common relevant allergens in patients with generalized dermatitis at our center in the urban midwestern US are quaternium 15/formaldehyde and bacitracin/neomycin. However, a large number of less common allergens account

TABLE 6.1 Guidelines for Patch Testing

Do	Don't
Place all indicated tests at one time	Conduct "screening" patch testing. Missed allergens may prevent cure
Use recommended concentrations and vehicles	Test patient's own products 'as is' unless intended for skin contact
Photo patch test sunscreens and photoactive fragrances and plants	Test only a standard series on patients with photo-distributed dermatitis
Interpret results 2–4 days and 4–7 days after placement	Interpret results immediately after removing patches
Become familiar with software and other resources to recommend alternatives	Discharge patients without extensive education and a list of alternatives to allergens
See patients for follow up 1 month after testing	Assume that positive patch tests are relevant to the patient's dermatitis

for the majority of cases, and it is useless to test only the most likely culprits. Without complete avoidance of all allergens, identification and avoidance of only one allergen will not lead to clinical improvement. Table 6.2 shows an example of a standard screening series for non-occupational dermatitis in the Midwestern United States.

Testing patients' personal care and occupational contactants "as is" can be helpful. However, results may be falsely negative due to insufficient concentration or bioavailability of the allergen from the product and a positive reaction does not pinpoint the culprit amongst several components. Positive reactions to items tested in non-standard dilution may also be irritant, and testing of healthy controls is required to interpret results.

Published literature regarding patch tests is complicated by the lack of standardized intervals for interpreting patch test results [5]. Although there is a standardized international grading system for the intensity of patch test response, the strength of the reaction varies with both the allergen and the number of days after application of the

TABLE 6.2 Example of a standard patch test series for non-occupational dermatitis in the Midwestern United States

Allergen	Common relevance
Preservatives:	Personal care products and biocides/disinfectants
2-Bromo-2-nitropropane-1,3,diol	"
2,5-Diazolidinylurea	"
Benzalkonium chloride	"
Benzyl alcohol	"
Benzoic acid/sodium benzoate	Food and cosmetics
Chloroxylenol (PCMX)	Personal care products and biocide/disinfectants
Chloromethylisothiazolinone/methylsiothiazolinone	"
DMDM hydantoin	"
Formaldehyde	"
Glutaraldehyde	"
Imidazolidinyl urea	"
Iodopropynyl butylcarbamate	"
Methyldibromo glutaronitrile/phenoxyethanol	"
Paraben mix	"
Triclosan	"
Quaternium-15	"
Fragrances	Personal care products and many other items
Balsam of Peru	and foods
Cinnamic aldehyde	and toothpaste
Fragrance mixes I and II	Personal care products
Tea tree oil	"natural" products
Ylang-Ylang oil	"

TABLE 6.2   (continued)

Allergen	Common relevance
Vanillin	and foods
Medicaments	Over-the-counter and prescription topical medications
Bacitracin	Antibiotic ointments
Benzocaine/dibucaine/lidocaine	Topical anesthetics
Budesonide	Fluorinated topical steroids
Clioquinol	Bag balm
Chlorhexidine	Antimicrobial
Di alpha tocopherol	Vitamin E
Neomycin	Antibiotic ointments
Tixocortol pivolate	Hydrocortisone group steroids
Triamcinolone acetonide	Topical steroid
Other components of personal care products and topical medicaments	
Amidoamine/cocamidopropyl betaine	Surfactants in shampoo/cleansers
Cocamide diethanolamide	and in coolants
Ethylenediamine dihydrochloride	Many industrial uses; in nystatin cream
Para-phenylenediamine	Hair dye
Glyceryl monothioglycolate	Hair permanent wave
Oxybenzone	Sunscreen
Propylene glycol	Solvent/humectant in personal care products, medicaments, foods, and coolant
Propolis (bee's glue)	Resin in personal care products/chewing gum

(continued)

TABLE 6.2   (continued)

Allergen	Common relevance
Sorbitan sesquioleate	Emulsifier
Stearyl alcohol	Lubricant, anti-foam agent
Wool wax alcohol (lanolin)	Ointments
Rubber chemicals	
Black rubber mix	Black and gray rubber
Carba mix/thiuram mix	Natural and synthetic rubbers
Mercapto mix	"
Mercaptobenzothiazole	and rust inhibitors
Thiourea	Neoprene
Metals	
Cobalt/Nickel	Steel
Potassium dichromate	Chrome and green cosmetics
Gold	Jewelry
Adhesives	
Butyl-phenol formaldehyde resin	Glue in shoes
Colophony	Pine resin/rosin/fragrance
Epoxy resin	Crafts/industry
Ethyl acrylate/methyl methacrylate	Bone cement/dentistry
2-Hydroxyethyl-methacrylate	Artificial nails
Ethyl cyanoacrylate	Liquid bandage
Tosylamide resin	Nail polish
Textile dyes and resins	
Dimethylol dihydroxyethyleneurea	Permanent press finish
Disperse Blue 106/124	Dark dyes for synthetics
Ethyleneurea, melamine formaldehyde mix	Permanent press for upholstery, etc.

patch tests, and these factors are often neglected in data analysis.

There is insufficient patient access for patch testing in the United States. The need for expertise in medical dermatology to identify the indication for patch testing combined with the required specialized knowledge of chemical sensitizers and resources to educate patients on alternatives create an insufficient supply of qualified providers.

Advocacy to change this unfortunate situation is limited by several factors: (1) Patients who are successfully patch tested are often cured, and they do not require support groups and other services of patient advocacy organizations. (2) The term dermatitis is used to indicate a variety of inflammatory skin disease which reduces public recognition. (3) Dermatitis is most often treated with generic medications and there has been little interest from the pharmaceutical industry in developing new treatments.

Diagnosis of Generalized Allergic Contact Dermatitis

Conducting patch tests is difficult with very little non-inflamed skin available. Figure 6.5 shows patch testing that is impossible to interpret due to dermatitis impinging on the patch test sites If the back and anterior thighs and upper arms are affected by dermatitis and there is no medical contra-indication, systemic corticosteroids can be used to suppress the dermatitis with patch test application planned immediately after the course is complete. A 10–14 day course is usually sufficient; dexamethasone may be a better choice than Prednisone if the patient is at risk for systemic contact dermatitis based on prior exposure to group A topical corticosteroids. Topical corticosteroids also will interfere with patch test results, and systemic therapy is generally preferred in these highly symptomatic patients.

Systemic corticosteroid treatment is particularly problematic when psoriasis is the unsuspected underlying dermatosis, as psoriasis often worsens after systemic corticosteroid treatment.

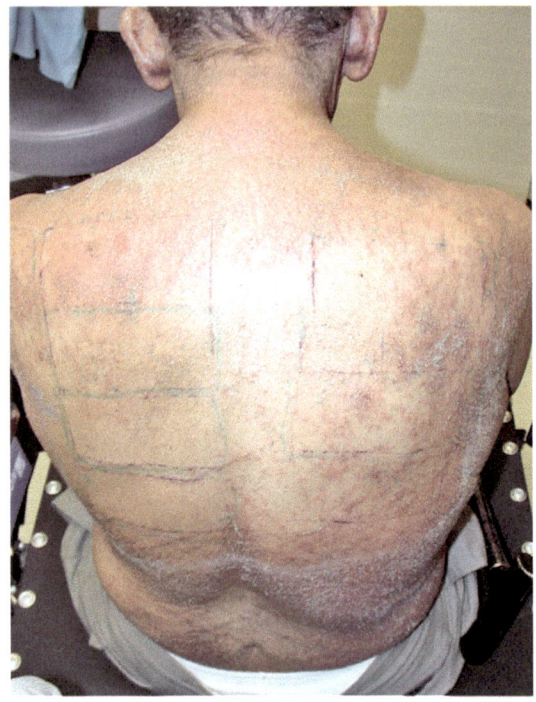

FIGURE 6.5 "Angry Back" with un-interpretable patch tests due to surrounding dermatitis impinging on the test site

A short (2–3 week) course of cyclosporine can be used to suppress inflammation in patients for whom corticosteroids are contraindicated, with testing performed immediately after completing the course. Systemic immunosuppressives prescribed for unrelated medical conditions such as rheumatoid arthritis should be discontinued for patch testing whenever possible. However, in some instances such as organ transplantation, these drugs cannot be discontinued.

Patch tests can sometimes produce strong reactions even in patients tested on immunosuppressants [6]. When patch tests are conducted during immunosupression, weak reactions (International Contact Dermatitis Research Group (ICDRG) grade of "?" denoting macular erythema) may be significant if there is a pattern of reaction to related antigens (e.g. several formaldehyde-releasing preservatives, or several corticosteroids, or several fragrances), or if there was high pre-test degree of suspicion, or if the reaction persists to day 7 after test placement.

After appropriate treatment of allergic contact dermatitis, skin biopsy is often more diagnostic of other dermatoses such as psoriasis.

Pre-test degree of suspicion for allergic contact dermatitis is usually lower with generalized than with localized dermatitis. However, entirely negative patch tests need to be considered with the same logic as in localized disease. That is, technical deficiencies in the test such as suppression of reaction by corticosteroid treatment could make the tests falsely negative. The culprit allergen may not have been tested, as in the patient in Fig. 6.2 with dermatitis to his hot tub additive when initially tested to a standard screening series. Testing to the patient's own products is important when evaluating negative patch tests in the setting of generalized dermatitis.

Repeat open application testing may be useful if clinical suspicion for allergy to a product is high but unconfirmed by patch tests, or if a patch test is suspected to be an irritant false positive. Exposure is dependent on both concentration of the allergen and time of exposure. For example, in rinse-off products patients may tolerate a known allergen. A study of MCI/MI allergic patients showed that at lower concentrations of allergen, repeat open application tests may take longer than 2 weeks to become positive [7].

Differential Diagnosis

Eczematous drug reactions and systemic contact dermatitis to components of medications are also in the differential diagnosis. Because patient recall for medications ingested intermittently is poor, it is useful to have the patient bring in the contents of their medicine cabinet. There is some literature regarding utility of patch tests for eczematous drug eruptions as well as for fixed drug eruption and pustular drug eruption.

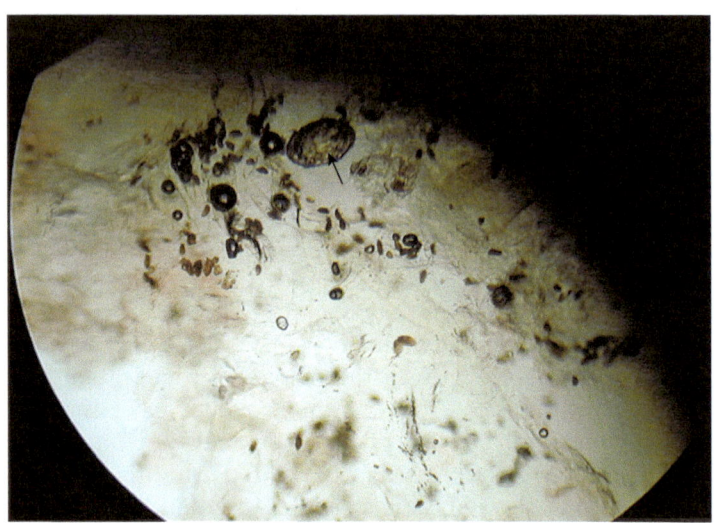

FIGURE 6.6 Scabietic egg (*arrow*) and feces

The sensitivity is less than 50% and tests are not standardized [8]. The diagnosis of eczematous drug eruption is usually confirmed by discontinuing the suspect medication for several weeks, but given the difficulty of pinpointing the culprit in patients taking many medications, patch testing is probably underutilized for this purpose.

Scabies: An Instructive Mimic

Scabies causes widespread dermatitis and is in fact a type of protein contact dermatitis. Despite the clues of facial sparing and flexural accentuation, the presentation is not that of papular urticaria as with other arthropod assaults, and the diagnosis is frequently missed. Multiple skin scraping can be required to confirm the diagnosis, and the microscopic examination is tedious. Figure 6.6 shows a scabietic egg and feces in a mineral oil preparation under light magnification. Hypersensitivity response to these components of the mite takes several weeks to resolve after the living mites are eradicated.

Scabies can be viewed as protein contact dermatitis. Scabies patients without a history of atopic dermatitis are more likely than healthy controls to have a positive atopy patch test to dust mite [9]. There is structural homology between house dust mites and scabies; the house dust mite atopy patch test is a crude extract from mites and feces. This also suggests that scabetic dermatitis patients are capable of reacting to protein on the skin. The many household contacts of scabies patients who are presumably infested but who do not itch may have immune systems incapable of the atopic-like ability to react to a protein antigen.

Other arthropod assaults such as cheyletiella mites from house pets may cause widespread papular urticaria that can mimic dermatitis [10], General veterinarians may miss the diagnosis of cheyletiella, and it is good practice to communicate this suspicion directly to the veterinarian as the diagnosis cannot be made by examination of the human patient alone.

References

1. Kagen MH, Wolf J, Scheman A, Nedorost S. Potassium peroxymonosulfate-induced contact dermatitis. Contact Dermatitis. 2004;51(2):89–90.
2. Rietschel R, Fowler J. Fisher's contact dermatitis. 6th ed. Hamilton: BC Decker; 2008.
3. Kanerva L, Elsner P, Wahlberg JE, Maibach HI. Handbook of occupational dermatology. Berlin: Springer; 2000.
4. Marks Jr J, Elsner P, DeLeo V. Contact and occupational dermatology. St. Louis: Mosby; 2002.
5. Cheng LS, Alikhan A, Maibach HI. Compilation of international standards for patch testing methodology and allergens. Dermatitis. 2009;20(5):257–60.
6. Rosmarin D, Gottlieb AB, Asarch A, Scheinman PL. Patch-testing while on systemic immunosuppressants. Dermatitis. 2009;20(5):265–70.

7. Zachariae C, Lerbaek A, McNamee PM, Gray JE, Wooder M, Menné T. An evaluation of dose/unit area and time as key factors influencing the elicitation capacity of methylchloroisothiazolinone/methylisothiazolinone (MCI/MI) in MCI/MI-allergic patients. Contact Dermatitis. 2006;55(3):160–6.
8. Barbaud A. Drug patch testing in systemic cutaneous drug allergy. Toxicology. 2005;209(2):209–16.
9. Ta kapan O, Harmanyeri Y. Atopy patch test reactions to house dust mites in patients with scabies. Acta Derm Venereol. 2005;85(2):123–5.
10. Rivers JK, Martin J, Pukay B. Walking dandruff and Cheyletiella dermatitis. J Am Acad Dermatol. 1986;15(5 Pt 2):1130–3.

Chapter 7
Systemic Contact Dermatitis

Key Concepts

- Systemic Contact Dermatitis is symmetrical, eczematous, and often urticarial
- Systemic challenge is best diagnostic test; patch testing is useful but not ideal
- Phenotypes of systemic contact dermatitis vary and may suggest the type of sensitizer

Definition

Systemic contact dermatitis means that cutaneous sensitization occurred and inflammatory cells subsequently home to the skin and sometimes other organs after exposure to the same or similar antigen by ingestion, inhalation, transcutaneous absorption, intravenous infusion, or implantation.

Systemic contact dermatitis may be viewed as a failure of tolerance. First exposure to an antigen via mucosa produces long-lasting tolerance; this is likely an evolutionary outcome to prevent food allergy. Mucosal surfaces are usually resistant to immune response even after the induction of cutaneous sensitization [1].

Systemic contact dermatitis often has both urticarial and eczematous features. Systemic reactions will often result in recall dermatitis at the relevant prior patch test site.

S.T. Nedorost, *Generalized Dermatitis in Clinical Practice,* 77
DOI 10.1007/978-1-4471-2897-7_7,
© Springer-Verlag London 2012

The variability of phenotypes of systemic contact dermatitis suggests that the phenotype depends on the immune mechanism involved in the initial cutaneous sensitization.

Mechanism of Systemic Contact Dermatitis

The exact mechanism and risk factors for induction of systemic contact dermatitis in humans are unknown. Involvement of both B and T cells is likely given the evidence suggesting a role for immunoglobulin in several types of systemic contact dermatitis.

Urticarial features, gastrointestinal symptoms, and a more rapid time course between exposure and reaction compared to cutaneous delayed type hypersensitivity are characteristic of systemic contact dermatitis.

The type I–type IV classification of immune reactions does not well describe mixed immune responses where antigen presentation is immunoglobulin assisted but cell-mediated.

As discussed in Chap. 4, atopic dermatitis can be considered a type of systemic contact dermatitis. Keratinocytes from inflamed skin of atopic dermatitis patients can take up antigen [2] and in a mouse model may function as antigen presenting cells leading to antigen-specific IgE production [3]. Systemic exposure can then cause immediate type hypersensitivity symptoms and dermatitis. Eosinophilic esophagitis is an antigen triggered mucosal reaction in atopic dermatitis patients often diagnosed by atopy patch tests to foods [4].

Special conditions are required for mucosal cells to develop an immune response to antigen. In the presence of all-*trans* retinoic acid, murine lymph nodes draining skin will behave like Peyer's patches draining small bowel and will produce B and T cells that home to the small intestine as well as to the skin [5]. The circumstances that allow such conditions are not defined, but systemic contact dermatitis to ingested antigen by definition must involve both cutaneous sensitization and a mucosal immune recognition.

Diagnosis of Systemic Contact Dermatitis

Antigen Presenting Cells in Skin Versus Other Mucosae

Patch testing is not an ideal method to diagnose systemic contact dermatitis. Although patch testing may reflect the circumstances of cutaneous sensitization, it is not reflective of antigen presentation via mucosa and T cell homing from these areas to skin.

Complexity of Food Chemistry and Absorption

Furthermore, dietary flavorants are chemically complex and use of screening allergy tests such as Balsam of Peru may not adequately screen for aromatics in food [6].

Even for metals, which may be absorbed without chemical change from the gastrointestinal tract, the amount delivered to skin may vary such that even oral challenge is not without confounders. Neils Veien, who has extensively studied vesicular hand dermatitis triggered by ingestion of metals, points out that the amount of dietary nickel transported to skin may depend on the time after ingestion, inter and intra-individual variation in absorption, influence of other dietary minerals on absorption, and concentration in perspiration leading to localization of dermatitis [6].

T Regulatory Subtypes and Migration Patterns

T regulatory cell dysfunction may play an important role in systemic contact dermatitis, yet this also may not affect patch test results. Mutations of the FoxP3 gene that eliminate CD4 + CD25+ naturally occurring T regulatory cells result in IPEX syndrome characterized by eczema and enteropathy. Type 1 regulatory T (Tr1) cells continue to function in IPEX [7], and in fact we have patch tested an IPEX patient to a

TABLE 7.1 Advice for patients regarding systemic contact dermatitis

Try 1 month of contact avoidance first; only a subset of patients with positive patch tests need to avoid systemic exposure

Removal of dental fillings, metallic plates, or devices is never a guarantee that symptoms will resolve

Threshold for reaction to ingested allergens may vary due to various factors affecting absorption

standard screening tray with entirely negative results (unpublished data). This suggests that Tr1 cells may be sufficient to suppress response to antigen in a patch test, but not to control enteropathy and dermatitis.

Patch testing is used as a proxy test in the absence of better understanding of the operative immunology.

As with conventional patch testing, allergens should be placed only on non-inflamed skin. For protein allergens, presentation on inflamed skin leads to sensitization, but repeated presentation on intact skin can induce cutaneous tolerance with increased IL-10 and antigen specific T reg cells even in sensitized mice [8]. This suggests a mechanism for reversal of systemic contact dermatitis that may be utilized therapeutically in the future.

In summary, patch testing can suggest an antigen that may be responsible for systemic contact dermatitis, but systemic avoidance and subsequent clinical improvement is required to confirm the diagnosis. Table 7.1 summarizes advice for patients with systemic contact dermatitis.

Clinical Clues to Systemic Contact Dermatitis

Contact Urticaria

Latex allergy was epidemic in the 1990s in health care workers, especially those with atopic dermatitis who often develop protein contact allergy. Type I symptoms

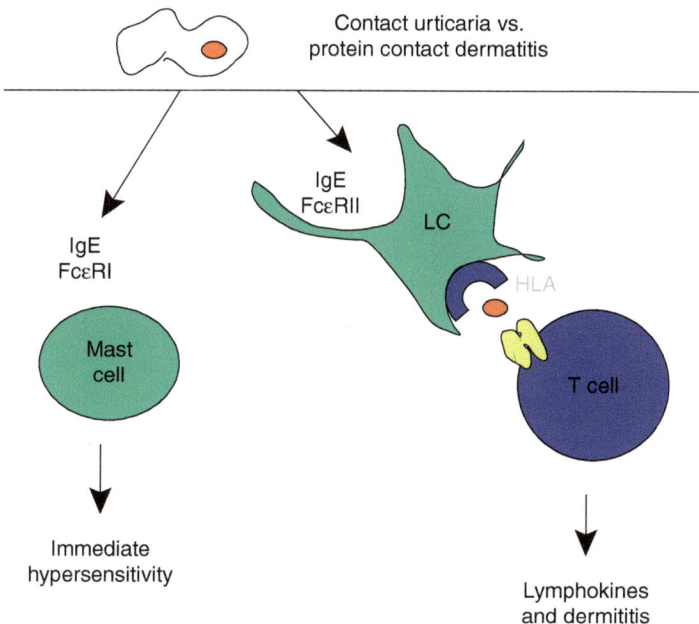

FIGURE 7.1 Schematic of immediate and delayed hypersensitivity reactions to proteins

predominated such as contact urticaria and anaphylactoid reactions [9]. Latex can also cause delayed type hypersensitivity associated with hand dermatitis [10] as well as the more common contact urticaria often associated with systemic symptoms. Figure 7.1 shows a simplified schematic of protein antigen triggering immediate and delayed reactions.

Atopic infants with food allergies often demonstrate contact urticaria as well as systemic reactions to foods such as milk, egg, and peanut. The type I reactions do not always occur in patients who demonstrate type IV reactions; this explains the need for atopy patch tests to diagnose dermatitis in addition to skin prick tests or serologic tests for antigen specific IgE to diagnose contact urticaria

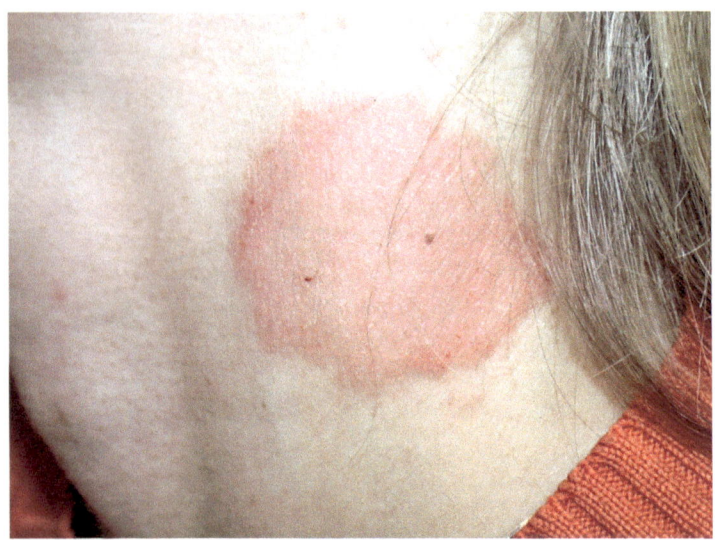

FIGURE 7.2 Allergic contact dermatitis site from medicament applied to an abrasion; site flared with subsequent ingestion of foods containing propylene glycol

Allergic Contact Recall: Ingestion Creates Dermatitis at Prior Patch Test Site

Systemic contact dermatitis to propolis, Balsam-related flavorants, compositae plants and herbals such as feverfew, and propylene glycol are the most common causes of systemic contact dermatitis detected by patch testing to a standard screening series. These components of food and medication are often applied to inflamed skin and may overcome previous oral tolerance resulting in systemic symptoms. Figure 7.2 shows propylene glycol induced recall dermatitis at the site of an abrasion which was treated with a medicament containing propylene glycol. Both these sites and the propylene glycol patch test site subsequently flared with ingestion of propylene glycol in foods and oral medications.

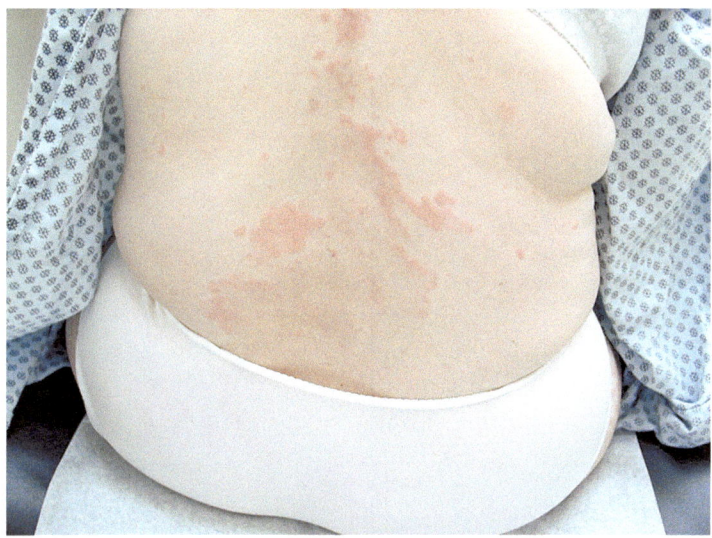

FIGURE 7.3 Systemic contact dermatitis to propolis; note the urticarial and eczematous morphologies

Mixed Urticarial and Eczematous Reactions

Figure 7.3 shows a reaction to oral propolis purchased from a health food store in a patient who had applied topicals containing propolis. The patient reacted within 24 h of ingesting the antigen. The rapidity of the reaction and urticarial features suggests a mixed immediate/delayed type mechanism.

Figure 7.4 shows systemic contact dermatitis with a positive patch test to Balsam of Peru that flared with ingestion of a nutritional supplement containing tomato.

Vesicular Hand Dermatitis (Dyshidrotic Eczema, Also Known as Pompholyx)

Vesicular hand dermatitis secondary to ingestion of metals can be experimentally reproduced [6]. There are also case reports

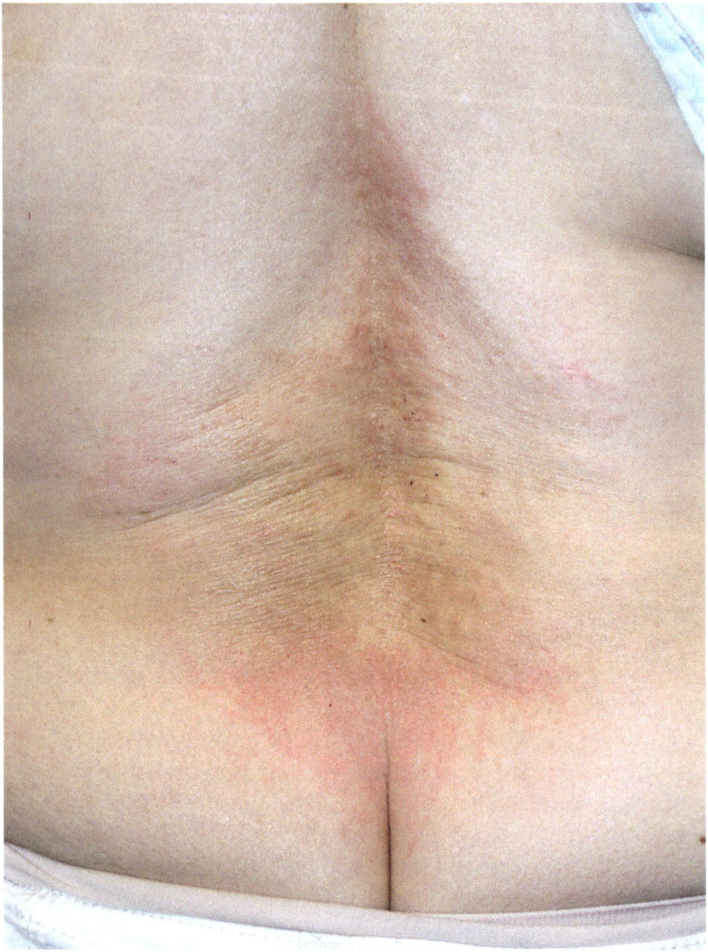

FIGURE 7.4 Systemic contact dermatitis triggered by tomato in a patient patch test positive to Balsam of Peru

of spontaneous appearance of vesicular hand dermatitis after infusion of intravenous immunoglobulin (IVIG) [11]. In one case, continued infusion of IVIG after onset of vesicular hand dermatitis induced baboon syndrome and then a maculopapular eruption [12]. This suggests that immunoglobulins also play a role in these types of systemic contact dermatitis.

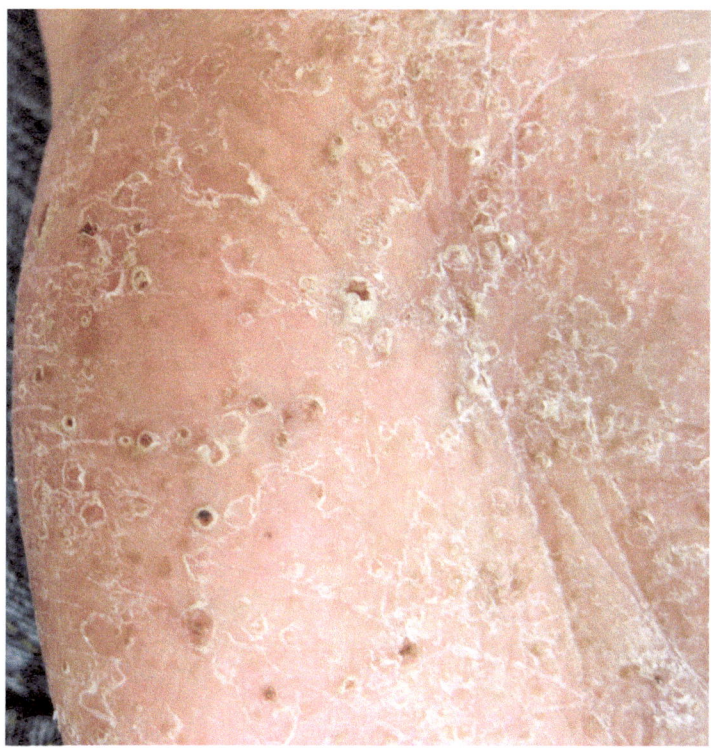

FIGURE 7.5 Dyshidrotic hand dermatitis presumably triggered by aeroallergen

Localization of vesicles to the hands and feet may be due to neuroimmune interactions unique to the hand and foot, as the disease process can be treated with neurotransmitter blockade [13, 14]. Substance P–releasing fibers are located with greatest density in the areas with greatest tactile sensation such as the palms and soles and are scanty elsewhere [15] Substance P is pro-inflammatory and agonists enhance induction of allergic contact dermatitis [16] while the substance P antagonist Spantide II diminishes allergic contact dermatitis [17, 18].

Figure 7.5 shows vesicular hand and foot dermatitis in a patient that occurred every spring, with or without handling plants in the garden. This suggests that aeroallergen exposure may trigger some cases.

Figure 7.6 (a)
Nickel allergic con-
tact dermatitis due
to snap on jeans.
(b, c) Same patient
as (a) with dys-
hidrotic hand and
foot dermatitis that
flared after inges-
tion of large quan-
tities of chocolate
covered nuts

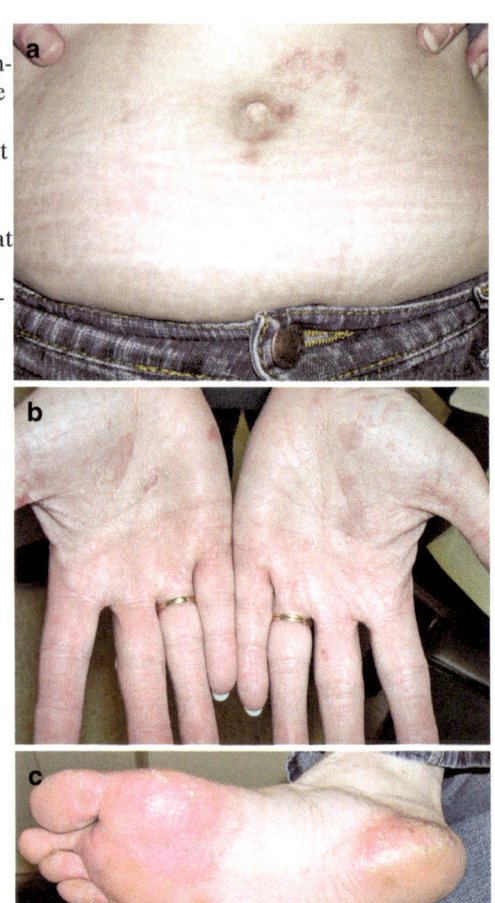

Figure 7.6 shows vesicular hand and foot dermatitis in a candy-maker who flared with ingestion of high nickel foods such as chocolate-covered nuts. Veien notes that only 10% of patients with a positive patch test to nickel benefit from dietary avoidance; he utilizes dietary nickel restriction only in patients with chronic vesicular hand dermatitis and intertriginous dermatitis, eyelid, or anogenital dermatitis and then usually only after confirmatory oral nickel challenge [6].

Dermatophyte infection of the feet can cause dyshidrotic hand eczema [19], another example of systemic contact

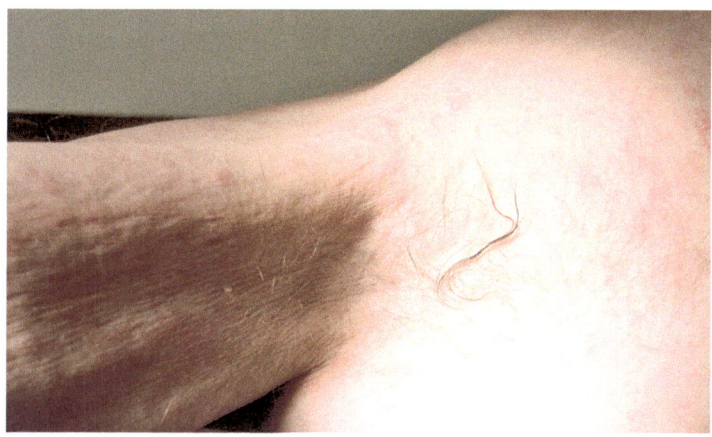

FIGURE 7.7 Eczematous drug eruption confirmed by re-challenge to glucosamine/chondroitin sulfate supplement

dermatitis due to a skin microorganism. This is also known as an 'id' reaction.

Baboon Syndrome

The immune mechanism of many drug reactions and systemic contact dermatitis due to drugs is poorly understood and the literature reflects this with descriptive phenotypes such as "baboon syndrome".

This sharply defined redness in the anogenital and other flexural areas, sometimes with pustules, was described in the 1980s due to exposure to mercury from broken thermometers and from ingestion of nickel and ampicillin. Many cases are due to initial exposure to a drug and have been renamed symmetrical drug-related intertriginous and flexural exanthema (SDRIFE) [20] to distinguish from allergic contact dermatitis syndrome due to previous contact sensitization with a drug [21].

Oral provocation testing is usually needed to confirm a systemic cause of SDRIFE; patch tests may be positive, but prick tests and lymphocyte transformation assays are usually negative [22]. Figure 7.7 shows an eczematous drug eruption most pronounced in the axillae that was confirmed with re-challenge to a glucosamine dietary supplement.

Erythema Multiforme

Erythema multiforme is a distinctive type of systemic contact dermatitis that may occur after allergic contact dermatitis to a strong sensitizer such as epoxy, para-phenylenediamine, or poison ivy [23]. As with other forms of systemic contact dermatitis, the immune mechanism is unclear but is known to involve immunoglobulin deposition and cytotoxicity presumably mediated by T cells [24]. Figure 7.8 shows a patient with erythema multiforme due to cutaneous exposure to epichlorhydrin, an epoxy intermediary.

Reaction to Implanted Devices

Metal on metal joint prostheses liberate metal particles and are associated with hypersensitivity reactions. Dermatitis and/or premature joint failure may occur. Dermatologists are often asked to perform patch testing either as a predictive test pre-operatively to assess risk of reaction or post-operatively in patients suspected of having an adverse event related to hypersensitivity. The validity of patch testing in these situations is not clear.

Pre-operative testing makes sense only if cutaneous sensitization explains reaction to implanted devices. If in fact positive patch tests can develop due to sensitization at the joint, then predictive testing may be flawed. If inflammation from joint pathology itself creates enough innate immune response to constitute danger signals, then sensitization may occur at the joint with the positive cutaneous patch tests a result rather than a cause [25].

Patient reported history of metal intolerance such as in jewelry does not correlate completely with patch test results to nickel. This may be because gold allergy explains some cases, but more likely is due to an immediate type response to metals, particularly in patients with pierced ears. In fact, exclusive B cell activation, rather than T cell activation, has been shown in some patients with hypersensitivity to metal joint prostheses [26]. If

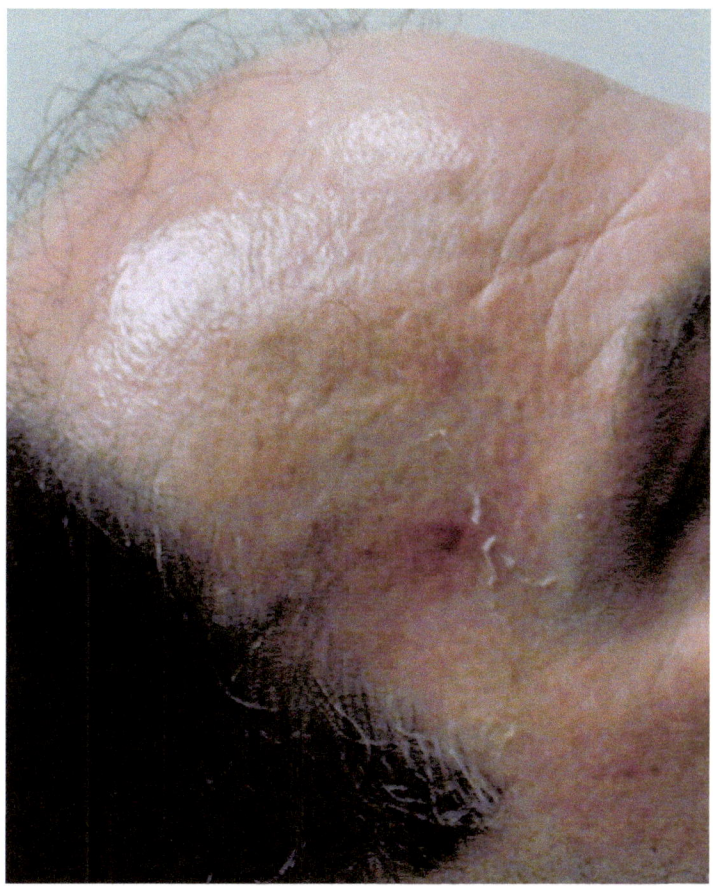

FIGURE 7.8 Erythema multiforme triggered by inhalation after occupational cutaneous sensitization to epichlorhydrin

systemic contact dermatitis is a mixed immediate/delayed type immune response, then patients who report a history of metal allergy and dyshidrotic eczema may be at the greatest risk for developing hypersensitivity to metals in implanted devices. This has not been studied, but given the questions about validity of patch tests in this setting, is recommended as a screening question until more robust data is published.

Dermatitis Herpetiformis: In Instructive Mimic

Dermatitis herpetiformis (DH) often mimics dermatitis clinically, but is characterized by IgA antibodies to gluten and a neutrophilic cutaneous infiltrate. DH and celiac disease share some features of systemic contact dermatitis in that they represent hypersensitivity to ingested gluten and can be cured by eliminating gluten in the diet.

Like atopic dermatitis, where early childhood exposure to infectious agents is protective (the hygiene hypothesis [27]) and caesarian rather than vaginal delivery increases the risk of respiratory atopy [28], celiac disease may be influenced by microbiome/immune interactions early in life. Children born by cesarean section are more likely to develop celiac disease later in life, perhaps due to defects in T regulatory cells and increased bowel permeability to proteins such as gluten [29].

Some patients with celiac disease have inflammatory cells homing to the skin, usually in extensor areas that may overexpress E-selectin in response to trauma. Even normal skin in DH patients over-expresses E-selectin in cutaneous endothelial cells, which may explain cutaneous homing of inflammatory cells [30].

DH can be considered an IgA- mediated form of systemic contact dermatitis due to gluten with its own unique pattern of expression.

References

1. Lencer WI, von Andrian UH. Elicitng mucosal immunity. N Engl J Med. 2011;365:1151–3.
2. Blume C, Foerster S, Gilles S, Becker WM, Ring J, Behrendt H, Petersen A, Traidl-Hoffmann C. Human epithelial cells of the respiratory tract and the skin differentially internalize grass pollen allergens. J Invest Dermatol. 2009;129(8):1935–44. Epub 2009 Feb 5.
3. Burns R, Luzina I, Nasir A, Haidaris CG, Barth RK, Gaspari AA. Keratinocyte-derived, CD80-mediated costimulation is associated with hapten-specific IgE production during contact

hypersensitivity to TH1 haptens. J Allergy Clin Immunol. 2005;115(2):383–90.

4. Spergel JM. Eosinophilic esophagitis in adults and children: evidence for a food allergy component in many patients. Curr Opin Allergy Clin Immunol. 2007;7(3):274–8.

5. Hammerschmidt SI, Friedrichsen M, Boelter J, Lyszkiewicz M, Kremmer E, Pabst O, Förster R. Retinoic acid induces homing of protective T and B cells to the gut after subcutaneous immunization in mice. J Clin Invest. 2011;121(8):3051–61.

6. Veien NK. Ingested food in systemic allergic contact dermatitis. Clin Dermatol. 1997;15(4):547–55.

7. Passerini L, Di Nunzio S, Gregori S, Gambineri E, Cecconi M, Seidel MG, Cazzola G, Perroni L, Tommasini A, Vignola S, Guidi L, Roncarolo MG, Bacchetta R. Functional type 1 regulatory T cells develop regardless of FOXP3 mutations in patients with IPEX syndrome. Eur J Immunol. 2011;41(4):1120–31. doi:10.1002/eji.201040909.

8. Dioszeghy V, Mondoulet L, Dhelft V, Ligouis M, Puteaux E, Benhamou PH, Dupont C. Epicutaneous immunotherapy results in rapid allergen uptake by dendritic cells through intact skin and downregulates the allergen-specific response in sensitized mice. J Immunol. 2011;186(10):5629–37.

9. Taylor JS, Praditsuwan P. Latex allergy. Review of 44 cases including outcome and frequent association with allergic hand eczema. Arch Dermatol. 1996;132(3):265–71.

10. Gottlöber P, Gall H, Peter RU. Allergic contact dermatitis from natural latex. Am J Contact Dermat. 2001;12(3):135–8.

11. Llombart M, García-Abujeta JL, Sánchez-Pérez RM, Hernando de Larramendi C. Pompholyx induced by intravenous immunoglobulin therapy. J Investig Allergol Clin Immunol. 2007;17(4): 277–8.

12. Barbaud A, Tréchot P, Granel F, Lonchamp P, Faure G, Schmutz JL, Béné MC. A baboon syndrome induced by intravenous human immunoglobulins: report of a case and immunological analysis. Dermatology. 1999;199(3):258–60.

13. Swartling C, Naver H, Lindberg M, Anveden I. Treatment of dyshidrotic hand dermatitis with intradermal botulinum toxin. J Am Acad Dermatol. 2002;47(5):667–71.

14. Klein AW. Treatment of dyshidrotic hand dermatitis with intradermal botulinum toxin. J Am Acad Dermatol. 2004;50:153–4.

15. Eedy DJ, Shaw C, Johnston CF, Buchanan KD. The regional distribution of neuropeptides in human skin as assessed by

radioimmunoassay and high-performance liquid chromatography. Clin Exp Dermatol. 1994;19(6):463–72.
16. Niizeki H, Kurimoto I, Streilein JW. A substance P agonist acts as an adjuvant to promote hapten-specific skin immunity. J Invest Dermatol. 1999;112:437–42.
17. Babu RJ, Kikwai L, Jaiani LT, et al. Percutaneous absorption and anti-inflammatory effect of a substance P receptor antagonist: spantide II. Pharm Res. 2004;21(1):108–13.
18. Scholzen TE, Steinhoff M, Bonaccorsi P, et al. Neutral endodpeptidase terminates substance P-induced inflammation in allergic contact dermatitis. J Immunol. 2001;166:1285–91.
19. Peck S. Epidermophytosis of the feet and epidermophytids of the hands: clinical, histologic, cultural, and experimental studies. Arch Dermatol Syph. 1930;20:44–76.
20. Häusermann P, Harr T, Bircher AJ. Baboon syndrome resulting from systemic drugs: is there strife between SDRIFE and allergic contact dermatitis syndrome? Contact Dermatitis. 2004;51 (5–6):297–310. Review.
21. Lachapelle JM. The spectrum of diseases for which patch testing is recommended. Patients who should be investigated. In: Lachapelle MJ, Maibach IH, editors. Patch testing/prick testing: a practical guide. Berlin: Springer; 2003, 189, p. 7–26.
22. Winnicki M, Shear NH. A systematic approach to systemic contact dermatitis and symmetric drug-related intertriginous and flexural exanthema (SDRIFE): a closer look at these conditions and an approach to intertriginous eruptions. Am J Clin Dermatol. 2011;12(3):171–80.
23. Wiedemeyer K, Enk A, Jappe U. Erythema multiforme following allergic contact dermatitis: case report and literature review. Acta Derm Venereol. 2007;87(6):559–61.
24. Bushkell LL, Mackel SE, Jordon RE. Erythema multiforme: direct immunoflourescence studies and detection of circulating immune complexes. J Invest Dermatol. 1980;74:372–4.
25. Schalock PC, Menné T, Johansen JD, Taylor JS, Maibach HI, Lidén C, Bruze M, Thyssen JP. Hypersensitivity reactions to metallic implants-diagnostic algorithm and suggested patch test series for clinical use. Contact Dermatitis. 2012;66:4–19. doi:10.1111/j.1600-0536.2011.01971.x.. Epub 2011 Sep 29.
26. Hallab NJ, Caicedo M, Epstein R, McAllister K, Jacobs JJ. In vitro reactivity to implant metals demonstrates a person-dependent association with both T-cell and B-cell activation. J Biomed Mater Res A. 2010;92(2):667–82.

27. Okada H, Kuhn C, Feillet H, Bach JF. The 'hygiene hypothesis' for autoimmune and allergic diseases: an update. Clin Exp Immunol. 2010;160(1):1–9.
28. Pistiner M, Gold DR, Abdulkerim H, Hoffman E, Celedón JC. Birth by cesarean section, allergic rhinitis, and allergic sensitization among children with a parental history of atopy. J Allergy Clin Immunol. 2008;122:274–9.
29. Decker E, Hornef M, Stockinger S. Cesarean delivery is associated with celiac disease but not inflammatory bowel disease in children. Gut Microbes. 2011;2(2):91–8.
30. Hall 3rd RP, Takeuchi F, Benbenisty KM, Streilein RD. Cutaneous endothelial cell activation in normal skin of patients with dermatitis herpetiformis associated with increased serum levels of IL-8, sE-Selectin, and TNF-alpha. J Invest Dermatol. 2006; 126(6):1331–7.

Chapter 8
Dermatitis Due to Systemic Disease

Key Concepts

- Myeloproliferative hyperesoinophilic syndrome presents with itch without rash and responds to imatinib
- Lymphocytic hypereosinophilic syndrome may present with urticaria, patchy dermatitis, or erythroderma and responds to corticosteroids or mepolizumab
- Dermatomyositis clinically resembles allergic contact dermatitis due to shampoo
- Cutaneous T cell lymphoma starts in photoprotected areas

Although hypersensitivity dermatitis can be associated with systemic symptoms, dermatitis can also be seen in systemic disease unrelated to allergy. This chapter deals with three systemic diseases that can present with generalized dermatitis. Immunodeficiency syndromes are also associated with generalized dermatitis and should be considered in patients with frequent or unusual infections.

Definition

Hypereosinophilic syndrome (HES) is defined by persistent eosinophilia ($>1.5 \times 10^9$/L on multiple occasions) without apparent cause and with evidence of end-organ damage. While any organ system can be affected, the most common are the heart, skin, lungs, and nervous system.

S.T. Nedorost, *Generalized Dermatitis in Clinical Practice,*
DOI 10.1007/978-1-4471-2897-7_8,
© Springer-Verlag London 2012

Types of HES

Myeloproliferative HES (M-HES) can present as generalized itch without primary skin lesions. Lymphocytic HES (L-HES) often presents as urticarial, eczematous, or erythrodermic disease. Patients may present with one or all of these symptoms at various times.

M-HES cases have features suggestive of an underlying myeloproliferative disorder causing hypereosinophilia. A subset of M-HES patients have a cryptogenic interstitial deletion on chromosome 4q12 that generates a fusion between the Fip1-like 1 (FIP1L1) and platelet derived growth factor receptor α (PDGFRA) genes resulting in the expression of a novel FIP1L1-PDGFRA (F/P) protein with constitutive tyrosine kinase (TK) activity. The abnormality is not detectable on routine karyotypes but is evident by FISH or RT-PCR analyses [1].

M-HES patients are corticosteroid resistant but respond to imatinib They exhibit elevated tryptase, normal IgE, anemia, myelofibrosis, hepatomegaly, and splenomegaly [2]. The most common complication in M- HES patients is endomyocardial fibrosis, and patients should be evaluated for cardiac involvement with an EKG, echocardiogram, or MRI [3].

Figure 8.1 shows a 70 year old woman with a 2 year history of intractable pruritus without any primary skin lesions. A bone marrow biopsy revealed FIP1L1/PDGFRA (F/P) fusion by FISH analysis. Oral imatinib was started with resolution of her symptoms.

L-HES patients have a subset of clonal Th-2 cells that overproduce IL-5, as well as IL-4, IL-13, and GM-CSF [4]. IL-5 promotes the differentiation and proliferation of eosinophils, while inhibiting eosinophil apoptosis peripherally IL-4, a cytokine which induces immunoglobulin class switching, is believed to account for the elevated levels of IgE and hypergammaglobulinemia seen in this population. In most cases the number of circulating T cells and their cytological phenotype are normal, therefore the gold-standard for L-HES diagnosis is based upon the measurement of the cytokine profile in the supernatants of *ex vivo* T cells [3].

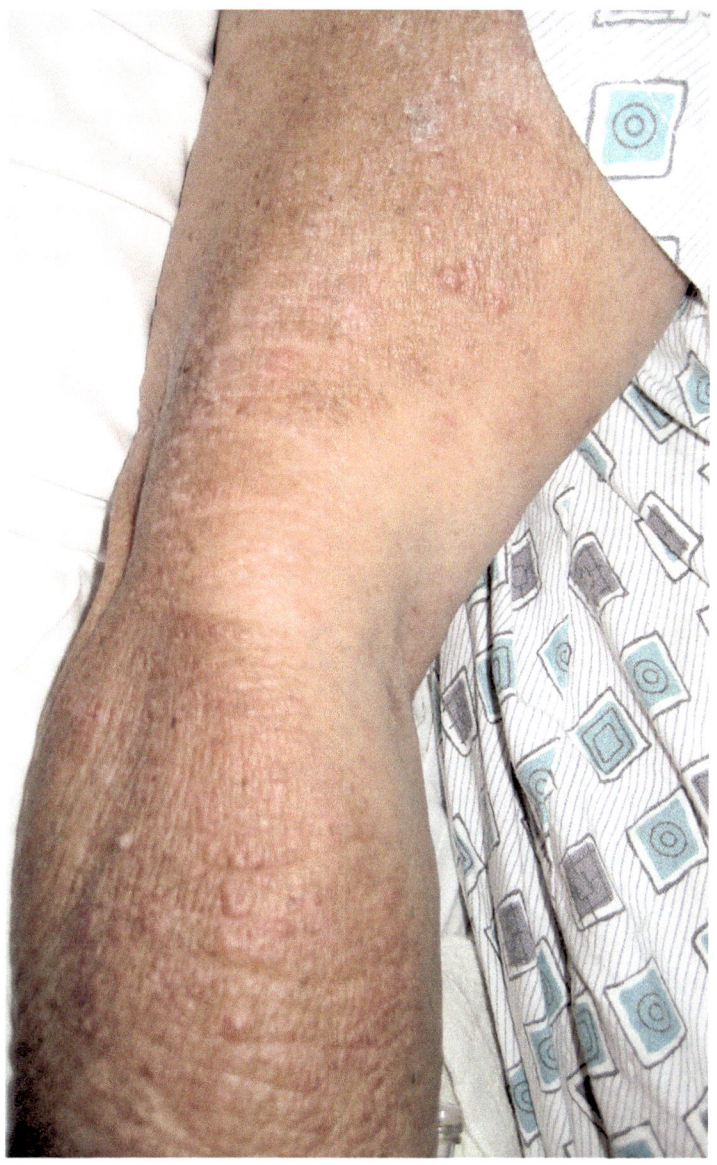

FIGURE 8.1 Myeloproliferative hypereosinophilic syndrome presenting as generalized itch; responsive to imatinib

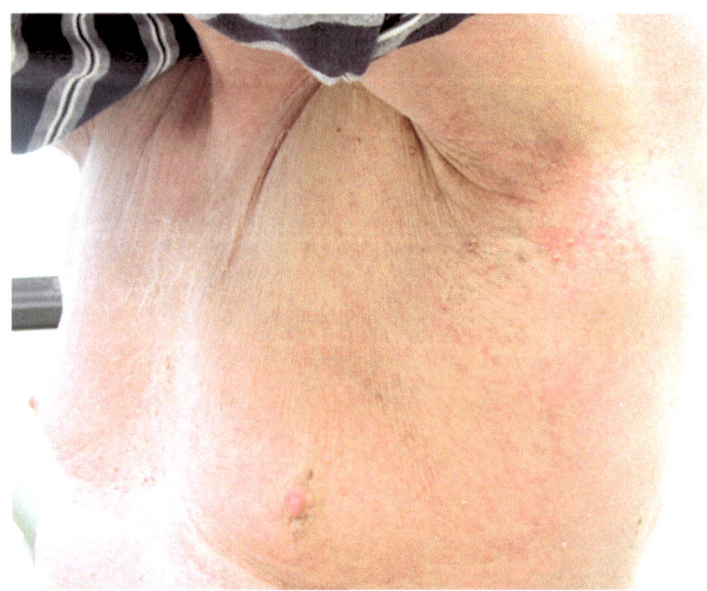

FIGURE 8.2 Lymphocytic hypereosinophilic syndrome fluctuating between patchy dermatitis and erythroderma

Skin biopsies typically show a perivascular infiltration of lymphocytes and eosinophils [4]. Due to the rarity of associated organ involvement in L-HES, cutaneous manifestations are considered a cardinal clinical feature of this disease [5] and explains why patients with HES seen in dermatology clinics predominantly have L-HES.

Corticosteroids are the mainstay of treatment in L-HES. Mepolizumab, a humanized anti-IL-5 monoclonal IgG antibody, has been shown to be effective as a corticosteroid-sparing agent [6].

Figure 8.2 shows a patient with a clonal T cell hypereosinophilia that fluctuated in intensity from patchy dermatitis to erythroderma.

Table 8.1 summarizes the distinctions between M-HES and L-HES.

TABLE 8.1 Comparison of types of HES

	M-HES	L-HES
Consider when hypereosinophilia and	Itch without rash	Urticaria and/or dermatitis
Check for	FIP1L1-PDGFRA mutation	T cell clone
May also see	Elevated tryptase and vitamin B12	Hypergammaglob-ulinemia
Watch for	Endomyocardial fibrosis	Lymphoma
Treat with	Imatinib	Corticosteroids or mepolizumab

Dermatomyositis

Dermatomyositis is the most eczematous of the connective tissue diseases. Because the face, scalp, eyelids, upper torso, and hands are often involved, the condition mimics allergic contact dermatitis such as to a hair product. Figures 8.3a, b shows a patient with dermatomyositis who was referred for evaluation of allergic contact dermatitis. The poikiloderma-tous sharply demarcated thin plaques on the torso and the periorbital lavender coloration and edema are characteristic.

Physical exam signs are important in establishing the diag-nosis, especially in patients without muscle symptoms. Because many dermatomyositis patients have a negative ANA, sero-logic studies are not useful when distinguishing dermatomyo-stis from dermatitis, although they may be useful to diagnosis systemic lupus. Itching with slight scale of the scalp, accentua-tion of the rash over knuckles and other bony prominences, and sparing of the interphalangeal skin that is involved in lupus are also helpful diagnostic signs.

Many patients such as the patient in Fig. 8.3 present to dermatologists with amyopathic dermatomyositis. The major-ity of these patients do not develop muscle or interstitial

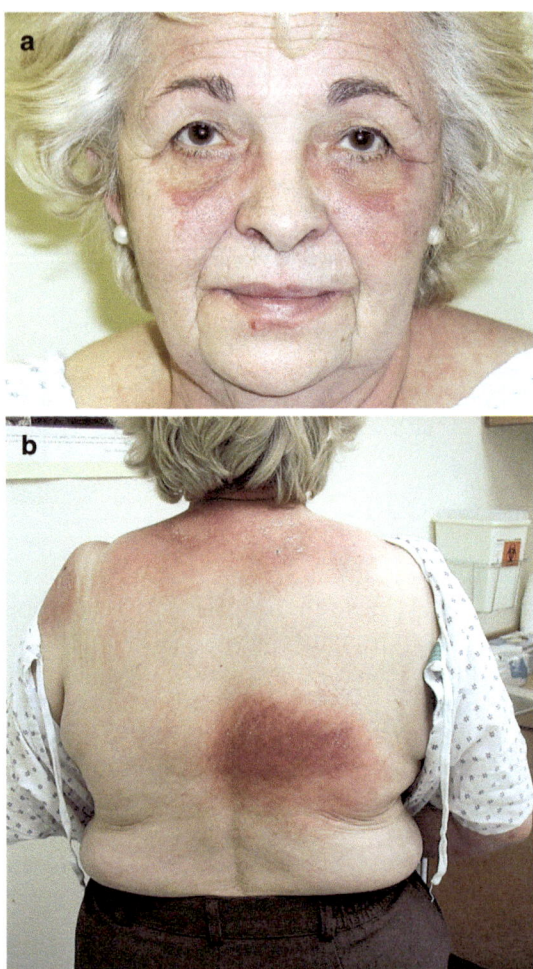

FIGURE 8.3 (**a**, **b**) Dermatomyositis patient referred with working diagnosis of allergic contact dermatitis; dermatomyositis can mimic allergy to hair products

lung disease and do not develop malignancy considered related to the diagnosis (within 3 years of diagnosis). Nevertheless, due to the association of malignancy with classic dermatomyositis with muscle involvement, thorough review of systems and physical exam with age-appropriate cancer screening is warranted [7].

Hydroxychloroquine is often effective for amyopathic dermatomyositis, but a significant percentage of patients develop a hypersensitivity rash [8]. This is an unusual adverse effect of hydroxychloroquine when used to treat lupus, and may lead to the diagnosis of dermatomyositis in a patient with previously undifferentiated connective tissue disease. A variety of immunosuppressives are used as corticosteroid sparing agents to treat resistant disease. Given the potential paraneoplastic nature of the disease, intravenous immunoglobulin (IVIG) is an effective and relatively safe, although very expensive, treatment option [9].

Cutaneous T Cell Lymphoma

Cutaneous T cell lymphoma (CTCL) of the classic type, also known as mycosis fungoides, is very indolent and often diagnosed as dermatitis for many years before the diagnosis of lymphoma is confirmed.

Initial lesions usually occur on photo-protected areas such as buttocks (see Fig. 8.4) or breasts. The lesions are often fairly sharply demarcated and may be irregularly pigmented, telangiectatic, and atrophic. Localized lesions may resemble nummular eczema. Multiple, excoriated lesions resemble patchy generalized dermatitis. Diagnosis may require more than one skin biopsy from untreated skin.

If extensive (>15% body surface area) cutaneous T cell lymphoma is diagnosed, or if there is palpable lymphadenopathy, CT scans of the chest, abdomen, and pelvis should be obtained to evaluate the patient for lymphadenopathy and hepatosplenomegaly. Additional work up should also include a lymph node biopsy if lymphadenopathy is detected.

Sezary syndrome is erythrodermic, advanced CTCL and can mimic erythrodermic dermatitis such as atopic dermatitis. Peripheral eosinophilia can be a clue, and special studies including flow cytometry for T cell markers and gene rearrangement to demonstrate clonality are helpful to support the diagnosis [10].

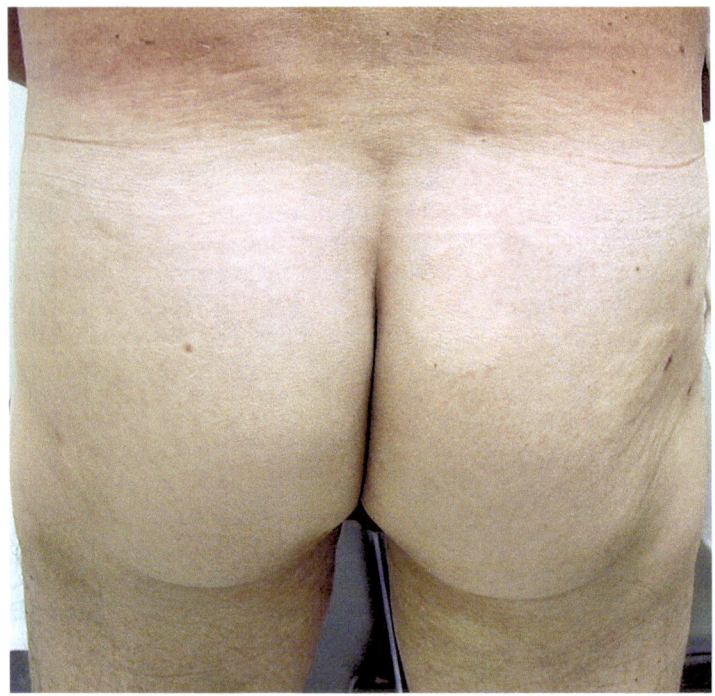

Figure 8.4 Cutaneous T cell lymphoma presenting with subtle, sharply demarcated plaques in a photo-protected site

Cutaneous T cell lymphoma can be treated with topical corticosteroids, nitrogen mustard, or retinoids or phototherapy in early stages. For more advanced disease, systemic retinoids, interferon alpha, IL-2 receptor fused to diphtheria toxin, and histone deacetylase inhibitors play a role for some patients [11].

References

1. Cools J, De Angelo DJ, Gotlib J, Stover EH, Legare RD, Cortes J, et al. A tyrosine kinase created by fusion of the PDGFRA and FIP1L1 genes as a therapeutic target of imatinib in idiopathic hypereosinophilic syndrome. N Engl J Med. 2003;348(13):1201–14.

2. Klion AD, Noel P, Akin C, Law MA, Gilliand DG, Cools J, et al. Elevated serum tryptase levels identify a subset of patients with a myeloproliferative variant of idiopathic hypereosinophilic syndrome associated with tissue fibrosis, poor prognosis, and imatinib responsiveness. Blood. 2003;101(12):4660–6.
3. Kahn JE, Bletry O, Guillevin L. Hypereosinophilic syndromes. Best Pract Res Clin Rheumatol. 2008;22(5):863–82.
4. Simon HU, Plotz SG, Dummer R, Blaser K. Abnormal clones of T cells producing interleukin-5 in idiopathic eosinophilia. N Engl J Med. 1999;341(15):1112–20.
5. Roufosse F, Cogan E, Goldman M. The hypereosinophilic syndrome revisited. Annu Rev Med. 2003;54:169–84.
6. Rothenberg ME, Klion AD, Roufosse FE, Kahn JE, Weller PF, Simon HU, et al. Treatment of patients with the hypereosinophilic syndrome with mepolizumab. N Engl J Med. 2008;358(12):1215–28.
7. Sontheimer RD. Clinically amyopathic dermatomyositis: what can we now tell our patients? Arch Dermatol. 2010;146(1):76–80.
8. Pelle MT, Callen JP. Adverse cutaneous reactions to hydroxychloroquine are more common in patients with dermatomyositis than in patients with cutaneous lupus erythematosus. Arch Dermatol. 2002;138(9):1231–3.
9. Callen JP, Wortmann RL. Dermatomyositis. Clin Dermatol. 2006;24(5):363–73.
10. Nagler AR, Samimi S, Schaffer A, Vittorio CC, Kim EJ, Rook AH. Peripheral blood findings in erythrodermic patients: Importance for the differential diagnosis of Sézary syndrome. J Am Acad Dermatol. 2012;66(3):503–8.
11. Prince HM, Whittaker S, Hoppe RT. How I treat mycosis fungoides and Sézary syndrome. Blood. 2009;114(20):4337–53.

Chapter 9
Diagnosis of Generalized Dermatitis

Key Concepts

- More than one diagnostic test is often required
- Repeat testing is sometimes required
- Diagnostic/therapeutic trials may be required to confirm diagnosis.

Initial Visit

The first step in diagnosis is to determine which disease processes are active. The subtypes of dermatitis (contact, atopic, stasis, systemic) often overlap, but keep in mind that they may also occur in conjunction with other processes. Dermatitis can occur in conjunction with the mimics discussed in earlier chapters.

Patient Education at Start of Visit

Allergic contact dermatitis may be a factor in any other form of dermatitis. Consideration of allergic contact dermatitis requires a solid partnership between the clinician asking thorough questions and the patient offering accurate answers. Before beginning the history, patients should understand the concept of delayed type hypersensitivity. Poison ivy is a useful example to relate the delay between exposure and symptom onset and the

S.T. Nedorost, *Generalized Dermatitis in Clinical Practice,*
DOI 10.1007/978-1-4471-2897-7_9,
© Springer-Verlag London 2012

prolonged period of symptoms from even a single exposure. Patients must also understand that a previous exposure could have initiated the dermatitis and that another allergen could perpetuate it, so that even past exposures need to be reported.

History and Exam

Ask where the rash began. Table 9.1 suggests most likely diagnoses based on initial location of the rash. In general, asymmetry favors external etiology (contact dermatitis) and generalized symmetrical dermatitis favors a systemic cause. However, there are some specific exogenous patterns that are symmetrical, such as textile dermatitis. Figure 9.1 demonstrates dermatitis in the posterior axillary line where perspiration and friction from clothing combine to accentuate textile-pattern dermatitis.

Pantomime is useful in asymmetrical dermatitis. For example, patients may use precise circular motions to apply medicament which can cause a sharply demarcated border that is otherwise unusual in contact dermatitis. Sparing of areas where patients cannot reach to apply personal care products is also suggestive of allergic contact dermatitis.

Look for primary lesions by asking the patient to point out a new lesion.

Note morphology. Table 9.2 suggests most likely diagnoses based on morphology.

List all personal care products, topical medicaments, and occupational/hobby exposures.

Inquire about affected family members, co-workers, and whether the patient sleeps with pets.

Obtain start dates and names of all medications, over-the counter drugs, and supplements.

Initial Tests

If the history suggests atopic dermatitis or if the patient has clinically impetiginized dermatitis, obtain a bacterial culture.

If the patient has facial sparing and flexural accentuation, scrape and examine a mineral oil preparation for scabies mites.

TABLE 9.1 Differential diagnosis of generalized dermatitis by site of initial involvement

Initial site of dermatitis	Leg (shin)	Head and neck	Interdigital hands, eyelids, or genitalia	Photo-distribution	Palmar /plantar	Fingertips /face	Textile pattern (axillary lines, neck)	Torso and extremities
Diagnostic considerations	*Child:* Atopic dermatitis due to shin guard occlusion	Allergic contact dermatitis	Irritant contact dermatitis	Photoallergic contact dermatitis	Psoriasis	Allergic contact dermatitis	Atopic dermatitis	Bullous disease
								Drug eruption
	Allergic contact dermatitis due to rubber	Atopic dermatitis	Scabies (not eyelids)	Photoallergic drug eruption	Allergic contact dermatitis		Allergic contact dermatitis	Cutaneous T cell lymphoma
							Dermato-graphism with excoriation	
	Adult: Stasis dermatitis with or without allergic contact dermatitis		Allergic contact dermatitis	Dermatomyositis				Systemic contact dermatitis

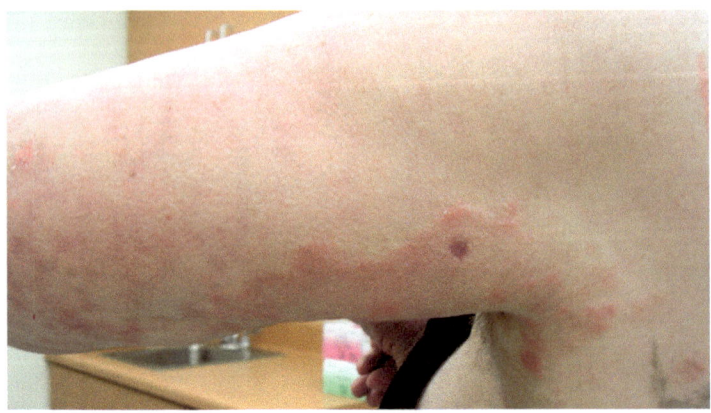

FIGURE 9.1 Textile allergic contact dermatitis localized to posterior axillary line

Skin biopsy is useful if bullous, papulosquamous, cutaneous T cell lymphoma or connective tissue disorders are in the differential diagnosis.

Blood count with differential to assess for eosinophilia may be useful if the patient is currently not on systemic corticosteroids.

Initial Plans and Preparation for the Second Visit

Discharge Patient Education

Patients need to understand that dermatitis is often multifactorial and therefore requires several concurrent interventions to relieve symptoms.

Diagnostic/Therapeutic Trials

Stasis dermatitis and irritant dermatitis are confirmed by therapeutic trial which should be initiated at this point. Gradient compression stockings for stasis dermatitis require

TABLE 9.2 Differential diagnosis of generalized dermatitis by additional morphologies noted on physical exam

Physical findings in addition to generalized dermatitis:	Vesicles on lateral fingers/palms	Urticaria	Itch disproportionate to rash	Sharp borders/well-delineated plaques
Diagnostic considerations	Systemic contact dermatitis to metals	Bullous pemphigoid	Current treatment obscuring disease	Psoriasis
	Bullous disease	Drug eruption	Scabies	Cutaneous T cell lymphoma
	Allergic contact dermatitis	Systemic contact dermatitis	Myelocytic hypereosinophilic syndrome	Dermatomyositis
		Scabies	Systemic disease causing itch e.g. lymphoma, biliary disease, renal disease, thyroid disease	
		Lymphocytic hypereosinophilic syndrome		
		Excoriated dermatographism from pressure urticaria		

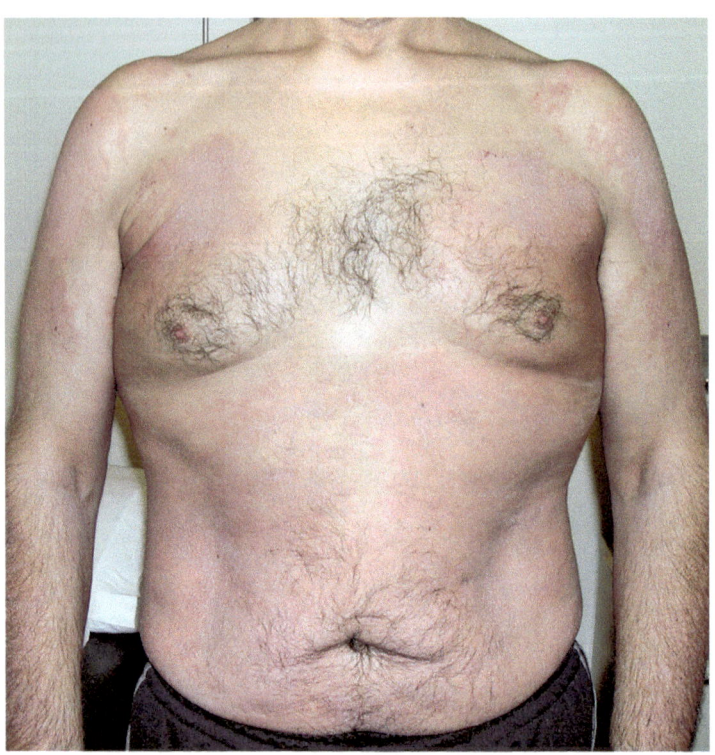

FIGURE 9.2 Atopic police officer with flare of dermatitis under an occlusive Kevlar vest

substantial planning and cooperation by the patient and family. Occlusive garments in atopic patients and other irritants such as excessive washing should be addressed at this time. Figure 9.2 shows an atopic police officer who improved with use of aluminum hexahydrate solution to reduce perspiration and absorbent powder containing clotrimazole applied under his occlusive bullet-proof vest. This regimen also improves shin guard dermatitis in atopic soccer players, although application will sting on inflamed skin.

If these therapeutic trials are insufficient, discuss plan with the patient for additional testing including patch testing and/or atopy patch testing.

TABLE 9.3 Short-term treatment to prepare patient for diagnostic testing

Barrier repair	Allergy	Infection control
Apply plain petroleum jelly immediately after bathing	Wash with unscented bar soap only	14 days of antibiotics aimed at staph aureus; bacterial culture
	Discontinue all previous topical personal care products and medicaments.	10 day course of systemic azole if adult atopic dermatitis is suspected
	10 days course of Prednisone up to 1 mg/kg/day OR if underlying psoriasis or medical contraindication 2–4 weeks of cyclosporine 3–5 mg/kg/day	

Plan for systemic immunosuppressives course to be complete just before patch tests are placed to reduce risk of generalized flare causing excited skin syndrome that interferes with patch test interpretation

Interval Treatment

For patients who have severe, generalized disease that is interfering with sleep and concentration, short-term systemic therapies may be needed to prepare the patient for further evaluation. Table 9.3 shows a treatment regimen intended only for short-term use between the initial consultation and the return visit for diagnostic testing approximately 2 weeks later. Diagnostic/therapeutic trials cannot be evaluated during systemic therapy, but may be started simultaneously and evaluated later.

Referral for Patch Testing

When considering patch testing, the practitioner should be equipped to test an extended standard series (usually 60–100 allergens) and additional allergens as suggested by occupational history and patterns noted on exam. If dermatitis is

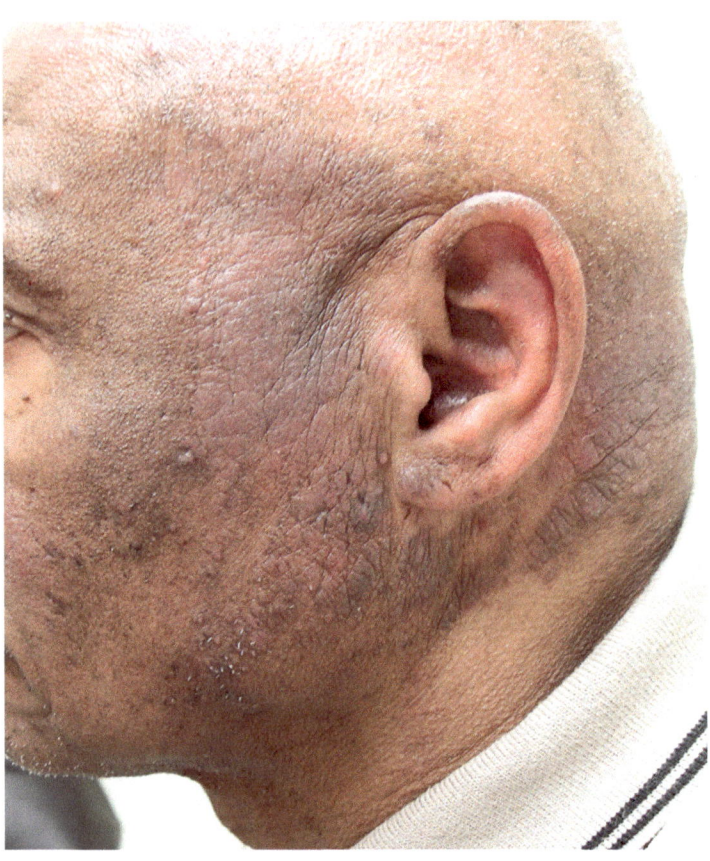

FIGURE 9.3 Actinic reticuloid; patient has positive photopatch tests

accentuated in photo-exposed areas, photo-patch testing is required. Figure 9.3 shows a patient with moderate control of actinic reticuloid on mycophenolate mofetil. Actinic reticuloid patients react to small amounts of ultraviolet light and have positive photo- patch tests to photo-sensitizers such as sunscreens. Adequate patch testing may require referral to a specialist dermatologist at an academic medical center if these resources are unavailable in the local community. Limited screening series are insensitive for diagnosis of allergic contact dermatitis. Incomplete diagnosis will not lead to cure and often discourages the patient from pursuing more thorough evaluation.

Evaluating Diagnostic Results

In uncomplicated cases, initial diagnostic maneuvers may lead to resolution of the dermatitis over several weeks. For example, compliance with gradient support stockings may resolve stasis dermatitis with autoeczematization.

Discontinuation of a systemic medication may resolve a drug eruption, although lichenoid reactions may take 3 months or more to resolve.

Treatment of a pet for cheyletiella may resolve the owner's dermatitis.

If the dermatitis is not resolved, proceed with patch testing, atopy patch testing and/or other appropriate tests (blood work, skin biopsy, mineral oil preparation) not obtained at the initial visit.

Patch test results must be evaluated first to distinguish irritant reactions from allergic results. This is done by assessing the patch test sites for morphology and strengthening or weakening of response between the first and second inspection of the sites (usually 3–4 and 5–7 days after patch test placement). Irritant (false-positive) patch tests have a high ratio of epidermal change to induration along with a weakening in the strength of the reaction between the first and second reading. Commonly, irritant results occur with non-standard allergens (i.e. testing personal care products as is), surfactants such as cocamidopropyl betaine, and metals such as potassium dichromate.

If the response is consistent with a true allergic reaction (Fig. 9.4), then the relevance must be assessed. Again, a poison ivy analogy may help the patient to understand the concept of irrelevant allergy. Explain that if poison ivy were tested, the patient would likely react, but that does not mean that poison ivy is causing the current dermatitis. The best test

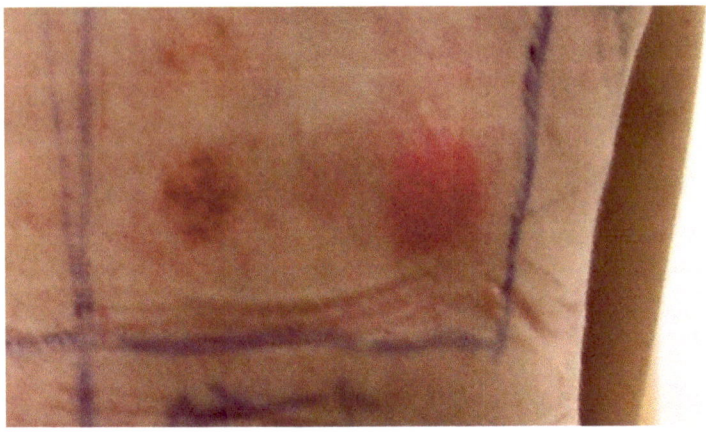

FIGURE 9.4 Irritant and allergic patch test reactions. Irritant reactions display epidermal discoloration and crusting (*left*); allergic reactions display induration due to dermal inflammation and may spread beyond the test chamber (*right*)

of relevance is complete avoidance of all allergens for 1 month with clearing, followed by flare of dermatitis when allergens are re-introduced either in open application tests or regular usage.

Patient Education

Complete avoidance is required! Patients must be provided with alternative products devoid of their allergen and cross-reacting components. The North American Contact Alternatives Group publishes resources for allergic patients that are posted on the American Contact Dermatitis Society website www.contactderm.org (membership required for database access).

Patients need to have plans to avoid allergens even outside their usual environment; they should travel with their own products and carry these products for use in public restrooms, etc.

One Month Follow Up After Patch Testing

If the dermatitis is less than 80% improved after the patch testing, consider the following:

1. Falsely negative patch tests due to technique. Was the patient off of systemic and topical immunosuppressives at the patch test site? Did the patches loosen?
2. Failure to test the offending allergen. Were the patient's own contactants tested at appropriate dilution?. DeGroot has written a helpful reference for determining best concentration and test vehicle [1].
3. Were potential photo-allergens exposed to 10 J of ultraviolet A light? Figure 9.3 shows lateral neck dermatitis with sparing of the submental skin seen in photoallergic contact dermatitis. This is most commonly due to sunscreen components in personal care products such as shampoo and moisturizers.
4. Exposure to a cross-reacting substance. Reviewing patient information handouts for cross-reactors and synonyms may help.
5. Retention of an allergen in clothing or gloves. Ointments are very difficult to remove completely from knit garments or inner glove surfaces.
6. Systemic contact dermatitis. Avoidance of the allergen in foods and medications may be required. This is most common with fragrances/flavorants and with propylene glycol.

Recalcitrant Generalized Dermatitis

Before considering chronic immunosuppressive therapies, reconsider all of the diagnostic possibilities. Figure 9.5 depicts a schematic diagnostic algorithm. Scabies, sub-bullous urticarial bullous pemphigoid, and cutaneous T cell lymphoma are all frequently missed on initial testing and may require one or more repeat tests to diagnose.

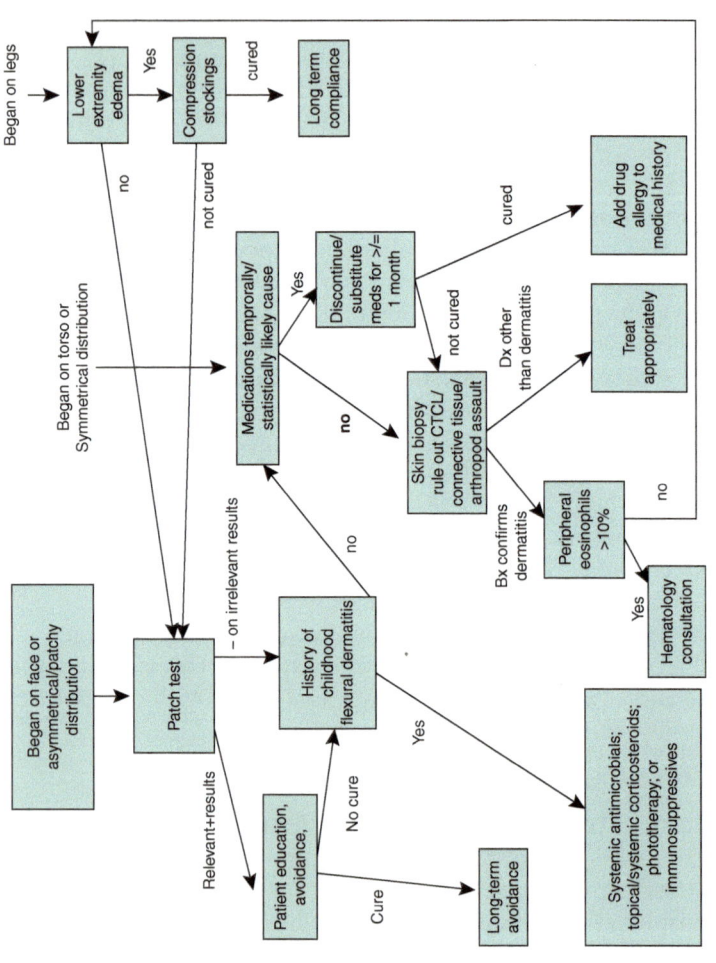

FIGURE 9.5 Diagnostic algorithm guided by initial site of dermatitis

Consider referral to a hematologist/oncologist for consideration of bone marrow biopsy if total eosinophils are persistently over 10% or if pruritus due to underlying hematological disease such as primary myelofibrosis is suspected [2].

Re-take the medication exposure history. Rarely, even intravenous exposures such as to hydroxyl ethyl starch volume expanders can lead to generalized itch beginning weeks after exposure and lasting for many months [3].

Consider referral to an interdisciplinary clinic (see Chap. 11) to support the patient in addressing simultaneous control of the skin barrier, allergen avoidance, infection, and stress as it is essential to address these simultaneously for dermatitis control.

References

1. De Groot AC. Patch testing. Test concentrations and vehicles for 4350 chemicals. 3rd ed. Wapserveen: Acdegroot publishing; 2008. 456 pp.
2. Vaa BE, Wolanskyj AP, Roeker L, Pardanani A, Lasho TL, Finke CM, Tefferi A. Pruritus in primary myelofibrosis: clinical and laboratory correlates. Am J Hematol. 2012;87:136–138.
3. Bork K. Pruritus precipitated by hydroxyethyl starch: a review. Br J Dermatol. 2005;152(1):3–12.

Chapter 10
Treatment of Generalized Dermatitis

Key Concepts

- Systemic treatment is often needed to prepare patients for diagnostic testing and for acute flares
- Maintenance treatment to prevent flares must address barrier dysfunction;, allergen avoidance, and infection control
- Prophylaxis against side effects should be addressed before beginning systemic therapies

Demands to Prescribe Systemic Therapy

Generalized dermatitis patients have severe pruritus which impairs quality of life.

Etiology is often difficult to determine, and many patients suffer for months without a definitive diagnosis. Physicians may respond by instituting systemic immunosuppressive therapy. Before resorting to chronic immunosuppression, exhaustive diagnostic work-up (see Chap. 9), a trial of non-immunosuppressive approaches (see Chaps. 3, 4, 5, 6 and 7), and prophylaxis against infections potentially due to immunosuppression should occur.

S.T. Nedorost, *Generalized Dermatitis in Clinical Practice,*   119
DOI 10.1007/978-1-4471-2897-7_10,
© Springer-Verlag London 2012

Short-Term Treatment
for Acute Flares: (Fig. 10.1)

Systemic treatments including antibiotics and rapidly-acting immunosuppressives such as Prednisone or cyclosporine may be used for short term treatment of disease flares or to prepare patients for patch testing (see Chap. 9 Table 9.3). For post-pubertal patients with atopic dermatitis, a 2 week course of systemic azoles to reduce Malasezzia colonization may improve head and neck dermatitis and can be prescribed with other systemic medications with caution to avoid drug interactions.

Systemic corticosteroids can interfere with growth in children, and have many adverse side effects. In atopic patients who are often of slight build, osteopenia is of special concern even in men [1]. Prophylactic treatment with bisphosphonates should be considered if systemic corticosteroids are used for more than 2 weeks [2] Cataracts are another adverse effect of corticosteroids of particular concern in atopic dermatitis, which is itself a risk factor for cataracts [3]. If systemic corticosteroid treatment is used, it is imperative to use the resulting clinical improvement as an opportunity to institute preventive strategies that may not otherwise be tolerated with inflamed skin. Treatment intervals of 2 weeks or less are preferred as there is no need for dosage tapering due to adrenal suppression.

Cyclosporine is useful in patients with dermatitis and psoriasis or patients who have a medical contraindication to systemic steroids. Cumulative life-time treatment should not exceed 6–12 months because of the risk of nephrotoxicity. Hypertension is a common side effect and may be worsened by magnesium wasting.

Wet wraps with hospitalization are an alternative for patients with acute flares who refuse or have medical contraindications to systemic treatments; improvement is noted within 3 days [4]. Because these also necessitate rest in an environment with reduced aeroallergens, it is difficult to differentiate the effect of the wet wraps from the effects of rest

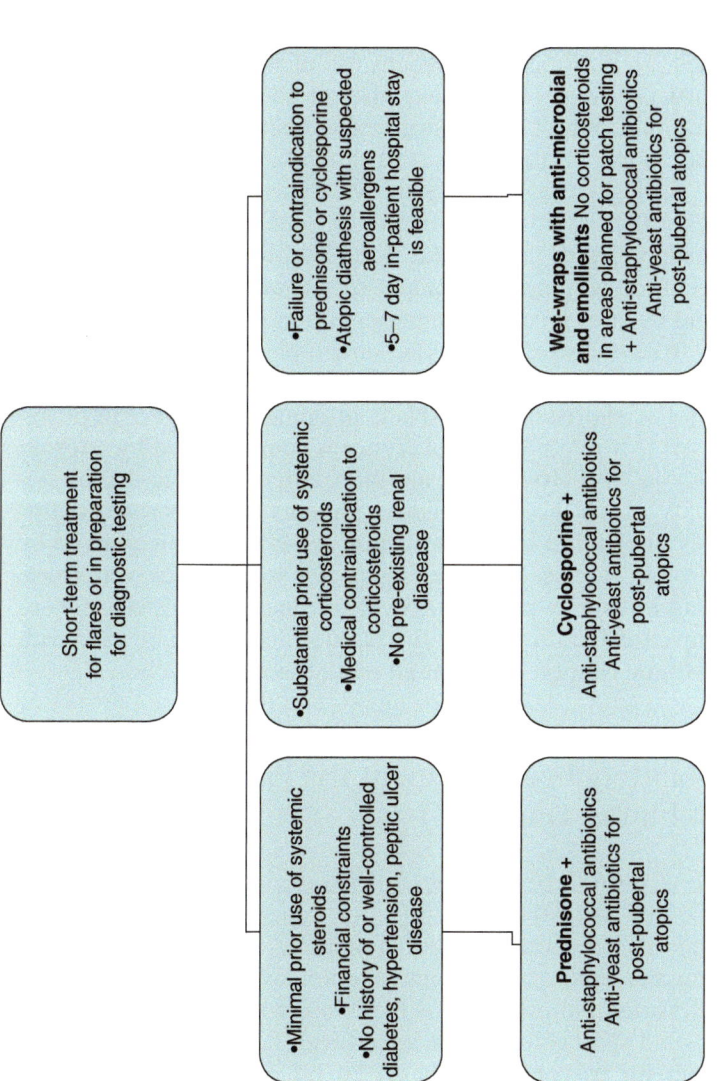

FIGURE 10.1 Short-term treatment algorithm for patients before diagnostic work-up

and reduced aeroallergen exposure. A German study demonstrated improvement in childhood atopic dermatitis with 3 days of wet wraps over chlorhexidine without corticosteroids [5]. Prolonged outpatient use of wet wraps over topical corticosteroids for 4 weeks offered no advantage compared to application of topical steroids without wet wraps, and there was an increased incidence of skin infections [6].

Topical corticosteroids are widely used for dermatitis and generally provide some degree of relief within days. Topical corticosteroids are useful for short-term flares, although attention to potential contact sensitization to either the steroid itself or inactive components is required.

In severely inflamed skin, some topical steroid is absorbed; with potent steroids this can suppress systemic cortisol levels [7]. For short-term use, this is insignificant and some physicians fear that patient adherence is compromised by "steroid phobia" [8]. However, even intermittent chronic use of steroids on the face or eyelids in patients with a rosacea diathesis can lead to steroid addiction syndrome, characterized by burning, redness, and swelling upon steroid withdrawal. These symptoms may persist for weeks or months and have severe impact on quality of life. Topical steroids should be used with extreme caution or not at all on the face and eyelids.

Maintenance Treatment for Prevention of Flares: (Fig. 10.2)

Long term dermatitis control requires attention to barrier, allergen avoidance, and infection control. Use of emollients and, if indicated, barrier creams or support stocking to enhance epidermal barrier function, avoidance of identified allergens, and prophylaxis to reduce cutaneous staphylococcal and yeast colonization are critical. Table 10.1 gives instructions for use of bleach baths for infection control. Because alkaline pH impairs barrier function [9], an acidic emollient should be applied immediately after bleach baths to enhance barrier repair.

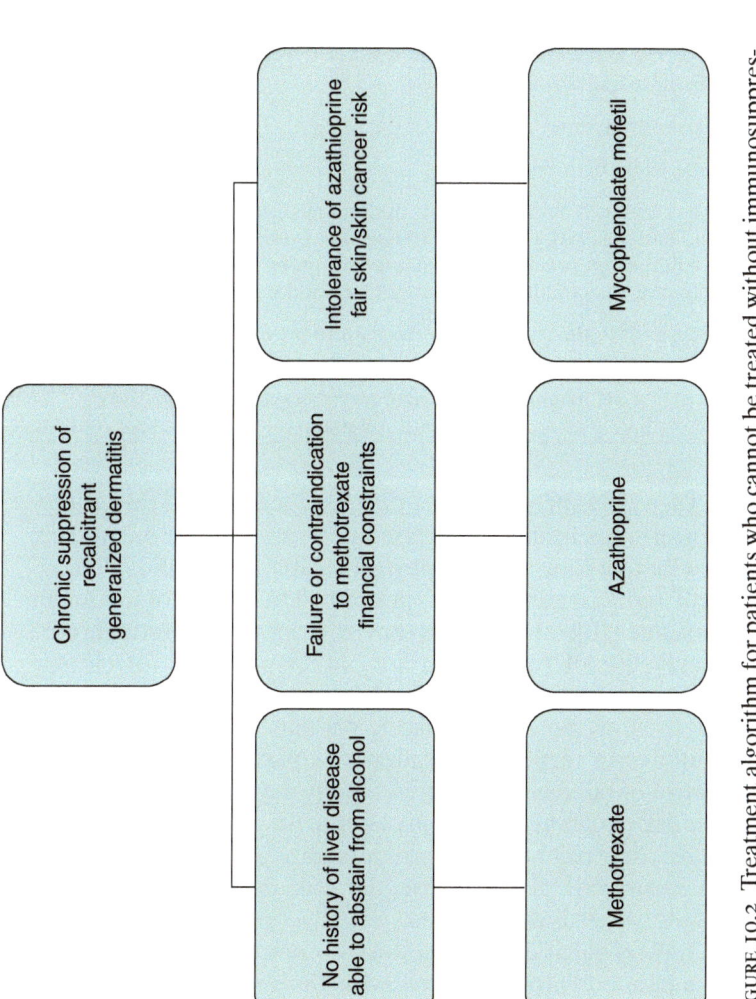

FIGURE 10.2 Treatment algorithm for patients who cannot be treated without immunosuppression despite thorough diagnostic evaluation

TABLE 10.1   Bleach baths for dermatitis

Swimming in a chlorinated pool can be substituted for a bleach bath.

1. Add about ½ cup of plain household bleach to the bathtub

2. Run the bathroom fan or open window to prevent irritation of the nose and throat

3. Soak for 10 min

4. Use white bath linens

5. Soak as much skin as possible; use antibacterial cleanser or shampoo with triclosan for areas that cannot be soaked. Children can practice blowing bubbles underwater (with adult supervision!) to allow exposure of face and scalp

6. Rinse off in the shower after the bath to prevent bleach residue from irritating skin

7. Apply a pH balanced moisturizer (such as acid mantle cream) immediately after rinsing, while still damp

There is controversy regarding long-term use of topical corticosteroids. Gradual reduction in efficacy may be due to lack of adherence or to tachyphylaxis. Although studies demonstrate reduced adherence to prescribed frequency of treatment over time [10], other studies show efficacy of intermittent twice weekly use of topical steroids for maintenance of chronic atopic dermatitis over a 16 week interval [11]. Cutaneous atrophy is rarely noted in pediatric patients, but elderly patients treated with regular application of topical corticosteroids for control of bullous pemphigoid rapidly develop severe atrophy. The risk of cutaneous atrophy later in life from chronic pediatric use of topical corticosteroids is unknown. Because topical corticosteroids also increase the risk of irritant dermatitis, long-term use is discouraged.

Topical calcineurin inhibitors do not cause tachyphylaxis or cutaneous atrophy. Even with the expected decrease in adherence over the first month of therapy, clinical improvement is noted [12]. However, both available formulations carry black box warnings regarding increased risk of malignancy. These are useful for treatment of eyelids and skin folds, but should be used with caution on sun-exposed skin until the risk of photocarcinogenesis is better defined.

Phototherapy is sometimes helpful in recalcitrant disease, but it is less beneficial than in psoriasis. Although ultraviolet B light is well known to interfere with allergic contact sensitization, and phototherapy may also benefit contact dermatitis by reducing effector response [13], there is no reason to use it in pure allergic contact dermatitis since avoidance is almost always preferable. In dermatitis with a mixed immune mechanism, phototherapy may be less effective than in pure T cell mediated processes. Phototherapy for atopic dermatitis may increase itch because perspiration from heat generated during phototherapy increases itching and scratching.

Vitamin D may be beneficial in atopic dermatitis, which may explain some of the benefit of phototherapy [14]. In mice, a vitamin D receptor agonist with weak calcium-mobilizing activity increased expression of genes associated with barrier function and anti-microbial peptides and increased T regulatory cells resulting in a decreased response to an ovalbumin patch test [15].

Long-Term Use of Immuosuppressives

When all other options have failed, it is sometimes necessary to treat with long-term use of steroid sparing agents. Comparative efficacy data is scarce and most of the studies enroll severely flared atopic dermatitis patients, such that improvement due to regression toward the mean complicates interpretation. A recent study showed both methotrexate 10–22.5 mg/week and azathioprine 1.5–2.5 mg/kg/day for 12 weeks were safe and effective [16]. Methotrexate works well for atopic dermatitis and dual-diagnoses such as psoriasis and bullous pemphigoid. [17]. Azathioprine or mycophenolate mofetil [18] are also effective; the latter is more expensive and carries a black box warning regarding progressive multifocal leukoencephalopathy, but has better gastrointestinal tolerance, Azathioprine may have higher likelihood of inducing cutaneous non-melanoma skin cancer in fair-skinned patients with long term use [19].

Prophylaxis for Infectious Complications

Screening for latent tuberculosis and viral hepatitis should occur before treatment begins. At least 2 weeks before initiating these treatments, the live vaccine for herpes varicella/zoster should be administered in previously unvaccinated children and in adults.

Pneuomococcal vaccine and seasonal influenza vaccine should also be up to date [20].

References

1. Haeck IM, Hamdy NA, Timmer-de Mik L, Lentjes EG, Verhaar HJ, Knol MJ, de Bruin-Weller MS, Bruijnzeel-Koomen CA. Low bone mineral density in adult patients with moderate to severe atopic dermatitis. Br J Dermatol. 2009;161(6):1248–54.
2. Furukawa F, Kaminaka C, Ikeda T, Kanazawa N, Yamamoto Y, Ohta C, Nishide T, Tsujioka K, Hattori M, Uede K, Hata M, Wakayama Study Group on Dermatological Use of Bisphosphonates. Preliminary study of etidronate for prevention of corticosteroid-induced osteoporosis caused by oral glucocorticoid therapy. Clin Exp Dermatol. 2011;36(2):165–8.
3. Bair B, Dodd J, Heidelberg K, Krach K. Cataracts in atopic dermatitis: a case presentation and review of the literature. Arch Dermatol. 2011;147(5):585–8.
4. Dabade TS, Davis DM, Wetter DA, Hand JL, McEvoy MT, Pittelkow MR, El-Azhary RA, Davis MD. Wet dressing therapy in conjunction with topical corticosteroids is effective for rapid control of severe pediatric atopic dermatitis: experience with 218 patients over 30 years at Mayo Clinic. J Am Acad Dermatol. 2012;67:100–106.
5. Abeck D, Brockow K, Mempel M, Fesq H, Ring J. Treatment of acute exacerbated atopic eczema with emollient-antiseptic preparations using the "wet wrap" ("wet pajama") technique. Hautarzt. 1999;50(6):418–21. German.

6. Hindley D, Galloway G, Murray J, Gardener L. A randomised study of "wet wraps" versus conventional treatment for atopic eczema. Arch Dis Child. 2006;91(2):164–8.

7. van Velsen SG, Haeck IM, Bruijnzeel-Koomen CA. Percutaneous absorption of potent topical corticosteroids in patients with severe atopic dermatitis. J Am Acad Dermatol. 2010;63-(5):911–3.

8. Aubert-Wastiaux H, Moret L, Le Rhun A, Fontenoy AM, Nguyen JM, Leux C, Misery L, Young P, Chastaing M, Danou N, Lombrail P, Boralevi F, Lacour JP, Mazereeuw-Hautier J, Stalder JF, Barbarot S. Topical corticosteroid phobia in atopic dermatitis: a study of its nature, origins and frequency. Br J Dermatol. 2011;165(4):808–14.

9. Cork MJ, Danby SG, Vasilopoulos Y, Hadgraft J, Lane ME, Moustafa M, Guy RH, Macgowan AL, Tazi-Ahnini R, Ward SJ. Epidermal barrier dysfunction in atopic dermatitis. J Invest Dermatol. 2009;129(8):1892–908.

10. Krejci-Manwaring J, Tusa MG, Carroll C, Camacho F, Kaur M, Carr D, Fleischer Jr AB, Balkrishnan R, Feldman SR. Stealth monitoring of adherence to topical medication: adherence is very poor in children with atopic dermatitis. J Am Acad Dermatol. 2007;56(2):211–6.

11. Glazenburg EJ, Wolkerstorfer A, Gerretsen AL, Mulder PG, Oranje AP. Efficacy and safety of fluticasone propionate 0.005% ointment in the long-term maintenance treatment of children with atopic dermatitis: differences between boys and girls? Pediatr Allergy Immunol. 2009;20(1):59–66.

12. Sagransky MJ, Yentzer BA, Williams LL, Clark AR, Taylor SL, Feldman SR. A randomized controlled pilot study of the effects of an extra office visit on adherence and outcomes in atopic dermatitis. Arch Dermatol. 2010;146(12):1428–30.

13. Schwarz A, Maeda A, Wild MK, Kernebeck K, Gross N, Aragane Y, Beissert S, Vestweber D, Schwarz T. Ultraviolet radiation-induced regulatory T cells not only inhibit the induction but can suppress the effector phase of contact hypersensitivity. J Immunol. 2004;172(2):1036–43.

14. Sidbury R, Sullivan AF, Thadhani RI, Camargo Jr CA. Randomized controlled trial of vitamin D supplementation for winter-related atopic dermatitis in Boston: a pilot study. Br J Dermatol. 2008;159(1):245–7.

15. Hartmann B, Riedel R, Jörss K, Loddenkemper C, Steinmeyer A, Zügel U, Babina M, Radbruch A, Worm M. Vitamin D

receptor activation improves allergen-triggered eczema in mice. J Invest Dermatol. 2012;132(2):330–6.

16. Schram ME, Roekevisch E, Leeflang MM, Bos JD, Schmitt J, Spuls PI. A randomized trial of methotrexate versus azathioprine for severe atopic eczema. J Allergy Clin Immunol. 2011;128(2):353–9.

17. Goujon C, Bérard F, Dahel K, et al. Methotrexate for the treatment of adult atopic dermatitis. Eur J Dermatol. 2006;16(2):155–8.

18. Neuber K, Schwartz I, Itschert G, Dieck AT. Treatment of atopic eczema with oral mycophenolate mofetil. Br J Dermatol. 2000;143(2):385–91.

19. Setshedi M, Epstein D, Winter TA, Myer L, Watermeyer G, Hift R. Use of thiopurines in the treatment of inflammatory bowel disease is associated with an increased risk of non-melanoma skin cancer in an at-risk population: a cohort study. J Gastroenterol Hepatol. 2012;27:385–9.

20. Glück T, Müller-Ladner U. Vaccination in patients with chronic rheumatic or autoimmune diseases. Clin Infect Dis. 2008;46(9): 1459–65. Review.

Chapter 11
Interdisciplinary Care for Dermatitis

Key Concepts

- Complex, multifactorial disease requires multiple interventions and interdisciplinary care
- Dermatology, psychology, allergy/immunology, dietetics, and nursing work together for dermatitis research and patient care
- Obstacles for interdisciplinary care of itch are similar to those for care of chronic pain

Patients hope for identification of a single triggering factor for their disease, and a prescription for a simple, curative medication. Because dermatitis is a multi-factorial disease, many patients cannot be cured and need to learn to manage multiple environmental interventions to control symptoms. For patients with moderate to severe dermatitis and/or difficult to manage dermatitis, interdisciplinary care may be helpful.

Interdisciplinary care that includes medical management, innovative diagnostics to determine environmental triggers, behavioral intervention, and patient education is expected to improve patient outcomes, and there is some published evidence to support this [1]. Educational sessions [2] and psychological support to help reduce scratching and improve sleep after disease flares are controlled are beneficial [3]. Habit reduction techniques to decrease scratching were synergistic when used with topical corticosteroids compared to benefit from the topical steroids alone [4].

S.T. Nedorost, *Generalized Dermatitis in Clinical Practice,*
DOI 10.1007/978-1-4471-2897-7_11,
© Springer-Verlag London 2012

Notably, psychological stress decreases barrier function in humans [5] and also increases susceptibility to cutaneous infections in mice [6] suggesting that stress reduction and relaxation techniques may impact pathophysiology.

Chronic itch is similar to pain in its impact on quality of life [7], but chronic pain has more commonly been addressed by interdisciplinary care. Interdisciplinary care for dermatitis shares the same obstacles as for pain. First, medicine in the US is organized by autonomous disciplines, and there is cultural change needed for providers to work collaboratively. Second, fee-for-service reimbursement creates incentive for providers to work independently, and does not discourage redundant effort. Thirdly, both patients and payers prefer attempts at cure to the effort required to manage disease through behavioral and educational interventions.

Quantitative evidence of value for interdisciplinary care for patients who cannot be cured by conventional care models may influence payers and improve patient access for these services. The current system of reimbursement does not support such innovation as most insurers will not pay for multiple providers to see a patient on the same day for the same diagnosis and will not reimburse the collaborative planning sessions that usually last about 15 min per dermatitis patient.

Future evaluation of interdisciplinary care and of new treatments will increasingly reflect the patient's perspective . Studies utilizing patient – centered data were recently published for use of alitretinoin in chronic hand dermatitis [8] and for patients with pruritus of various causes [9].

Our interdisciplinary clinic starts with an educational session that acquaints patients with diagnostic techniques, mind-body connections, and the treatments appropriate for both acute flares and for maintenance. Patients complete a preference for treatment form (Table 11.1) that is used in creating a treatment plan. Patient preference for participation in medical decision making is inversely correlated with adherence to asthma treatment [10], and we hope that soliciting patient preferences in creating a treatment plan will lead to improved adherence to that plan.

TABLE 11.1 What will you do to manage your eczema?

	Barrier	Allergy	Infection
For flares	Wet wraps	Short course of steroid pills	Antibiotic pills
	Apply ointments immediately after bathing	Immunosuppressive pills (transplant medications)	
		Apply topical steroids or non-steroid immunosuppressives	
For prevention	Apply creams or lotions immediately after bathing	Avoid skin contact with allergens identified by patch testing	Swim in chlorinated pool 3× weekly
	Apply barrier creams to block allergens in the air like pollen	Modify diet to avoid allergens identified by skin prick or patch testing	Bleach baths 3× weekly
	Mind-body work to reduce scratching	Mind-body work to reduce itching	Use of medicated shampoo and body wash

Circle all items that you are willing to consider if recommended by your health care providers. Choose one or more item from each column

Use this form to write down questions that may help you to decide

After the group education session led by a dermatology nurse, patients are evaluated by an allergist for triggers of immediate hypersensitivity symptoms including oral allergy syndrome, contact urticaria, asthma, and allergic rhinitis. A dermatologist evaluates for irritant and allergic contact dermatitis and for the presence of skin disease in addition to dermatitis. A psychologist assesses and teaches biofeedback, habit reduction, and refers for psychotherapy as needed. A dietician assists with food avoidance strategies.

A potential pitfall of interdisciplinary care is that hand-offs increase the risk of missing an important step in the sequence of care. Table 11.2 is a sample check-list of actions that are often needed in the management of generalized dermatitis.

The interdisciplinary clinic also creates opportunities for research in diagnostic techniques and in methods of health care delivery for this medically complex disease.

Likewise, interdisciplinary basic science research will benefit our understanding of dermatitis.

An example of interdisciplinary research translating to interprofessional care is the recognition of the importance of biofilms in atopic dermatitis. Advances in genomics have increased our appreciation of biofilms on the skin. Biofilms are communities of microorganisms in a polymeric matrix. Atopic dermatitis patients have a biofilm containing colonies of staphylococcal aureus. Epidermal cells and staphylococci likely contribute glycoproteins to this biofilm that disappears with processing for routine histology [11]. Biofilms in atopic dermatitis make staphylococci very difficult to eradicate, in part by reducing polymorphonuclear phagocytosis of individual bacteria which results in production of increased quantities of inflammatory cytokines that contribute to chronic inflammation [12].

Biofilms on oral mucosa are better studied than those on skin, and keratin is part of the oral biofilm structure [13]; barrier function is abnormal allowing penetration of antigens, but not invasion as would be seen in the complete absence of epithelial barrier. Barrier defects in atopic dermatitis may

TABLE 11.2 Checklist for interdisciplinary dermatitis clinic patient visits

	Check if completed
Diagnosis of dermatitis verified by dermatologist examination	
Patient education on role of barrier, infection, and allergy	
Thorough history and exam to determine need for patch testing	
Treatment of infection and plan for prophylaxis	
Emollients selected with consideration of patient preference	
Control of lower extremity edema if indicated	
Allergens and replacement alternatives identified	
Medications prescribed for treatment of acute flares	
Mind-body work for habit reduction and to alleviate stress	
Follow up to detect errors in physician diagnosis or patient adherence	
If inadequate response, re-consideration of mimics of dermatitis	
If still inadequate response, discussion of risks and benefits of systemic maintenance treatments	

predispose to the formation of biofilms that differ from those in non-atopic patients. In fact, oral disease may be more common in atopic children. In the 2007 National Survey of Children's Health, parents of children with severe atopic dermatitis were significantly more likely to report symptoms of 'bleeding gums' or 'toothache' than in children without atopic dermatitis [14].

Generalized dermatitis is multi-factorial and associated with both cutaneous and extra-cutaneous morbidities. The burden of dermatitis is significant both in symptoms of itch and pain and in emotional distress due to disruption of sleep, concentration, and ability to work. Interdisciplinary clinical and research efforts offer hope for patients with complex medical disease, and dermatitis should be no exception.

References

1. Chou JS, Lebovidge J, Timmons K, Elverson W, Morrill J, Schneider LC. Predictors of clinical success in a multidisciplinary model of atopic dermatitis treatment. Allergy Asthma Proc. 2011;32(5):377–83.
2. Staab D, Diepgen TL, Fartasch M, Kupfer J, Lob-Corzilius T, Ring J, Scheewe S, Scheidt R, Schmid-Ott G, Schnopp C, Szczepanski R, Werfel T, Wittenmeier M, Wahn U, Gieler U. Age related, structured educational programmes for the management of atopic dermatitis in children and adolescents: multicentre, randomised controlled trial. BMJ. 2006;332(7547):933–8.
3. Kelsay K, Klinnert M, Bender B. Addressing psychosocial aspects of atopic dermatitis. Immunol Allergy Clin North Am. 2010;30(3):385–96.
4. Norén P, Melin L. The effect of combined topical steroids and habit-reversal treatment in patients with atopic dermatitis. Br J Dermatol. 1989;121(3):359–66.
5. Garg A, Chren MM, Sands LP, Matsui MS, Marenus KD, Feingold KR, Elias PM. Psychological stress perturbs epidermal permeability barrier homeostasis: implications for the pathogenesis of stress-associated skin disorders. Arch Dermatol. 2001;137(1):53–9.
6. Aberg KM, Radek KA, Choi EH, Kim DK, Demerjian M, Hupe M, et al. Psychological stress downregulates epidermal antimicrobial peptide expression and increases severity of cutaneous infections in mice. J Clin Invest. 2007;117:3339–49.
7. Kini SP, DeLong LK, Veledar E, McKenzie-Brown AM, Schaufele M, Chen SC. The impact of pruritus on quality of life: the skin equivalent of pain. Arch Dermatol. 2011;147(10):1153–6.

8. Blome C, Maares J, Diepgen T, Jeffrustenbach S, Augustin M. Measurement of patient-relevant benefits in the treatment of chronic hand eczema–a novel approach. Contact Dermatitis. 2009;61(1):39–45.

9. Blome C, Augustin M, Siepmann D, Phan NQ, Rustenbach SJ, Ständer S. Measuring patient-relevant benefits in pruritus treatment: development and validation of a specific outcomes tool. Br J Dermatol. 2009;161(5):1143–8.

10. Schneider A, Wensing M, Quinzler R, Bieber C, Szecsenyi J. Higher preference for participation in treatment decisions is associated with lower medication adherence in asthma patients. Patient Educ Couns. 2007;67(1–2):57–62.

11. Akiyama H, Hamada T, Huh WK, Yamasaki O, Oono T, Fujimoto W, Iwatsuki K. Confocal laser scanning microscopic observation of glycocalyx production by Staphylococcus aureus in skin lesions of bullous impetigo, atopic dermatitis and pemphigus foliaceus. Br J Dermatol. 2003;148(3):526–32.

12. Vlassova N, Han A, Zenilman JM, James G, Lazarus GS. New horizons for cutaneous microbiology: the role of biofilms in dermatological disease. Br J Dermatol. 2011;165(4):751–9.

13. Dongari-Bagtzoglou A, Kashleva H, Dwivedi P, Diaz P, Vasilakos J. Characterization of mucosal Candida albicans biofilms. PLoS One. 2009;4(11):e7967.

14. Silverberg JI, Simpson EL. Eczema severity is associated with multiple comorbid conditions and increased healthcare utilization. Poster 260. Presented at the Society for Investigative Dermatology Annual Meeting, Raleigh, May 2012.

Glossary

Adaptive immune system The portion of the immune system consisting of antibody responses and cell-mediated responses, with B and T lymphocytes as effector cells, respectively. This system recognizes specific pathogens (antigens) and creates immunological memory after an initial response to a specific pathogen, leading to an enhanced response to subsequent encounters with that same pathogen.

Aluminum hexahydrate Antiperspirant that is applied to the skin. Also has broadly anti-microbial properties [HSlzle E, Neubert U Antimicrobial Effects of an Antiperspirant Formulation Containing Aqueous Aluminum Chloride Hexahydrate Arch Dermatol Res (1982) 272:321 329]

Antigen A substance identified by cells in the immune system as being foreign to the body; initiates and mediates the production of an antibody or cell mediated response by the adaptive immune system.

Atopic (atopy) A genetically predisposed, clinical hypersensitivity state with allergy against common environmental protein antigens, most commonly manifested as allergic rhinitis, asthma or atopic dermatitis.

Atopy patch test A type of patch test done in atopic dermatitis patients by applying protein allergens usually used to elicit standard IgE-dependent reactions when tested by skin-prick test.

Balsam of Peru Aromatic resin of trees grown in Central America used as a flavoring and fragrance in many products and also found in topical medicaments. It contains a mixture of many substances that are generally related to cinnamon, vanilla, and clove.

Benzyl alcohol An aromatic alcohol used as a preservative, solvent and anesthetic. It is also used in photographic development, perfumes, the food industry, and pharmaceuticals and cosmetics as a bacteriostatic.

Bullous pemphigoid An acquired autoimmune blistering disease in which autoantibodies are directed against components of the basement membrane zone of the skin. Typically, bullous pemphigoid occurs in elderly persons with a flexural distribution of skin lesions. The blister formation may be preceded by an urticarial or eczematous rash.

Ceramide A major lipid constituent of lamellar sheets in the stratum corneum composed of sphingosine and a fatty acid. Ceramides plays an essential role in maintaining the water permeability and barrier function of the skin.

Cetyl/stearyl alcohol A mixture of fatty alcohol used as an emulsion stabilizer, foam boosting surfactant, and aqueous and non-aqueous viscosity-increasing agent. It is widely used in cosmetics and personal care products.

Cheyletiella A genus of mites, also known as walking dandruff mites. Cheyletiella can infest dogs, cats, and other animals and cause dermatitis in humans.

Cocamidopropyl betaine A surfactant derived from coconut oil and dimethylaminopropylamine, used in shampoos, bath gels, bar soaps, and liquid soaps and cosmetics. It is commonly used in "no tears" types of shampoos. It may be used for thickening, foam stabilizing, or anti-static.

Cocamide DEA A coconut derived ingredient often used as a cleanser, foaming agent, thickener, or stabilizer in shampoos and soaps. It is also used in cosmetics, industrial cooling lubricants and hydraulic fluids.

Colophony Also known as rosin, is extracted from the sap of different species of conifers such as pine and spruce trees. Three types of colophony (gum, wood, and tall oil) are distinguished depending on the method of extraction. It is used in a wide variety of products for its ability to make things sticky and to increase water resistance of paper. Colophony may be found in adhesives, adhesive tapes, polishes, waxes, cosmetics, chewing gums, and topical medications.

Commensal A relationship in which one organism liveses on or within another organism and derives benefit without harming or benefiting the host.

Compositae A large family of plants containing the potential allergens *sesquiterpene lactones*. Some well-known examples are daisy, chrysanthemum, sunflower, dandelion, lettuces and ragweed. Botanical extracts from some of these are added to skin and hair products.

Conventional patch test A method used to determine if a specific substance causes allergic reaction of the skin via a type IV or delayed type hypersensitivity reaction. During patch testing, small amounts of allergen are placed onto discs mounted on hypoallergenic tape and then placed on the back for 48 h

Cutaneous lymphocyte antigen A cell surface protein that is expressed by T cells and is a receptor for the vascular lectin endothelial cell-leukocyte adhesion molecule 1. CLA expression plays an important role in migration of T cells to the skin.

Dermatophyte A group of fungi that cause infections of the skin, hair and nails due to their ability to obtain nutrients from keratinized material. Infections caused by these fungi are also known by the names "tinea" and "ringworm." Toenail and fingernail infections are referred to as onychomycosis.

Dermatitis herpetiformis A autoimmune blistering skin disease characterized by intensely itchy, chronic papulovesicular eruptions, usually on the extensor surfaces of the elbows knees, buttocks, and back. Patients are hypersensitive to gluten and may have a gluten-sensitive enteropathy (celiac sprue disease) in the small bowel.

Dyshidrotic eczema Also known as pompholyx, is a chronic, and recurrent eruption characterized by small vesicles on the palms, soles, and/or lateral aspects of the fingers. It can be associated with atopic dermatitis, contact dermatitis and fungal infection. Ingestion of metal ions, emotional stress and smoking are aggravating factors.

Erythema multiforme A hypersensitivity reaction that occurs in response to medications, infections or illness. It is characterized by the appearance of target-like lesions on the skin. There may be mucous membrane involvement. Necrotic keratinocytes are noted on histology.

Filaggrin A filament-associated protein that binds to keratin filaments. It is vital for keratinocytes to mature properly into flat corneocytes that form the outermost protective layer of our skin (cornified cell envelope). It plays an important role in forming a functional barrier by limiting water loss and preventing entry of chemicals and infectious agents into the epidermis.

FISH analysis Fluorescent *in situ* hybridization is a cytogenetic technique used to detect and localize the presence or absence of specific DNA sequences on chromosomes. It is done using a fluorescent probe that binds to certain specific chromosomes.

Fc receptor A protein found on the surface of certain cells of the immune system such as macrophages, neutrophils and mast cells. Fc receptors bind to antibodies which are attached to infected cells or pathogens or antigens. This stimulates phagocytic or cytotoxic cells to destroy microbes or infected cells and may initiate an allergic response.

GM-CSF Granulocyte-macrophage colony-stimulating factor is a cytokine that stimulates stem cells to produce granulocytes (neutrophils, eosinophils and basophils) and monocytes. GM-CSF also has functions such as activation and recruitment of inflammatory cells including neutrophils and eosinophils, and enhances the effector functions of neutrophils and macrophages.

Group A corticosteroids A group of corticosteroids known as hydrocortisone type in which there is no substitution on the D ring except a short-chain ester on C21 or a thioester on C21. Corticosteroids are divided into four classes, based on chemical structure. Allergic reactions to a member of a class typically indicate an intolerance of the others of that class. This group includes hydrocortisones, hydrocortisone acetate, cortisone acetate, tixocortol pivalate, predniso-lone, methylprednisolone and prednisone.

Habit reduction A way to change an acquired behavior that has become almost involuntary as a result of frequent rep-etition. For example, it has been postulated that scratching becomes a habit in atopic eczema patients.

IL-4 A type of cytokine produced by activated T lympho-cytes, mast cells basophils and eosinophils. It has many biological roles, including the stimulation of activated B-cell and T-cell proliferation, and the differentiation of precursor T helper cells to the Th2 subset that mediates humoral immunity and modulates antibody production.

IL-5 A cytokine produced by T helper-2 cells and mast cells that functions as a growth and differentiation factor for both B cells and eosinophils. It is also a main regulator of eosinophil activation and increased immunoglobulin secre-tion. The increased production of this cytokine is reported to be related to asthma or hypereosinophilic syndromes.

IL-10 A cytokine produced by monocytes and lymphocytes that functions as an important regulator of the immune system. This cytokine has anti-inflammatory effects by inhibiting synthesis of pro-inflammatory cytokines such as IFN-γ, IL-2, IL-3, TNF-α and GM-CSF. It also enhances antibody production and suppresses the antigen-presenta-tion capacity of antigen presenting cells.

IL-13 A cytokine produced primarily by activated Th2 cells involved in B-cell maturation and differentiation. This cytokine down-regulates macrophage activity, thereby inhibiting the production of pro-inflammatory cytokines and chemokines. This cytokine is found to be critical to the pathogenesis of allergen-induced asthma but operates through mechanisms independent of IgE and eosinophils. Most of the biological effects of IL-13 are similar to those of IL-4 but are less important given the more potent role of IL-4.

Imatinib A 2-phenylaminopyrimidine derivative that functions as a specific inhibitor of tyrosine kinase enzymes. It is used to treat certain types of leukemia and other cancers of the blood cells, gastrointestinal stromal tumors, dermatofibrosarcoma protuberans, hypereosinophilic syndrome and AIDS-related Kaposi's sarcoma. It works by blocking the abnormal protein that signals cancer cells to multiply.

Induration A condition of being hardened; a palpable raised hardened area of the skin.

Innate immune system Also known as non-specific immune system or the first line of defense. This system functions by identifying and eliminating pathogens that might cause infection with immediate maximal response but no immunologic memory. Innate systems of defense include natural anatomic barriers, the complement system and IL-1, and cells including NK cells, neutrophils and macrophages.

Interdisciplinary care A health care system in which a group of health care and heath care-related professionals from different disciplines work together. Teams are made up of a variety of providers such as dietitians, physiotherapists, social workers, primary care and specialist physicians, nurse practitioners, and others. Team members consistently collaborate to solve patient problems that are too complex to be solved by one discipline or many disciplines in sequence.

International Contact Dermatitis Research Group (ICDRG) grading scale A system for clinical scoring of allergic patch test reactions.

$-$ = Negative reaction;

? = Doubtful reaction: erythema only, no infiltration;

+ = Weak positive reaction: redness, induration, and possibly papules;

+ + = Positive reaction: erythema, induration, papules, and vesicles;

+ + + = Strong positive reaction: intense erythema, induration, and coalescing vesicles.

IPEX syndrome **I**mmune dysregulation, **p**olyendocrinopathy, **e**nteropathy **X**-linked syndrome is caused by mutations in the *FOXP3* gene, which results in the absence or dysfunction of regulatory T cells. Presentation is most commonly with the clinical triad of watery diarrhea, eczematous dermatitis, and endocrinopathy (most commonly insulin-dependent diabetes mellitus) beginning in the first year of life.

Keratinocytes The predominant cells in the epidermis. The primary function of keratinocytes is the formation of a barrier against pathogens and environments such as heat, UV radiation and water loss. They produce keratin (a protein that provides strength to skin, hair, and nails) during the process of differentiation into the dead and keratinized cells of the stratum corneum. Immunologic functions of keratinocytes are increasingly recognized.

Langerhans cells Dendritic cells of the skin and mucosa which contain large granules called Birbeck granules. Langerhans cells are found principally in the epidermis. They function as antigen-presenting cells which bind, uptake and process antigens and transport them to the lymph nodes, eventuating in cell-mediated immune reactions.

Lichenoid drug eruption A drug eruption resembling lichen planus characterized by violaceous, papular, often polygonal, pruritic lesions. However, lichenoid drug eruptions tends to have more confluent areas and less mucosal involvement than idiopathic lichen planus. The eruption often appears weeks or months following ingestion, contact, or inhalation of certain agents such as gold salts, beta blockers, antimalarials, thiazide diuretics and penicillamine.

Lyocell A cellulose fiber made from wood pulp. The fiber is produced by a solvent spinning technique, and the cellulose undergoes no significant chemical change. Lyocell fibers are soft, absorbent, very strong when wet or dry, and resistant to wrinkles. It is commonly found in women's clothing and bandages and protective suiting material.

Methylchloroisothiazolinone/methylisothiazolinone (MCI/MI) Preservatives with antibacterial and antifungal properties. They are known as the registered trade name Kathon CG when used in combination. MCI/MI are found in many water-based personal care, household, and industrial products.

Microbiome The collection of microbes (bacterial, fungal, viral), their genetic elements (genomes) and environmental interactions in a defined environment.

Multidisciplinary care A type of care relating to use of several disciplines at once. Refers to doctors who specialize in different medical areas working together to provide a comprehensive treatment plan for their patients. Differs from interdisciplinary care in that there is less collaborative interaction between the specialists, with patients interacting with multiple specialists within the same venue or health system

Nummular dermatitis A form of dermatitis, also known as discoid dermatitis. It is characterized by round-to-oval erythematous plaques most commonly found on the legs and buttocks. It is commonly found in people in their 60s and flare-ups are associated with dry skin.

Pantomime Expression by gestures without speech. Useful to understand how patients interact with materials that may cause allergic contact dermatitis

Papulosquamous A condition characterized by papules and scaling on the surface. Examples of papulosquamous disease include psoriasis, pityriasis rosea, and lichen planus.

Phenotype The observable physical or biochemical characteristics of an organism, as determined by both genetics and environmental influences.

Photoallergy A delayed hypersensitivity reaction requiring ultraviolet activation of the chemical substance to which the individual has become sensitized.

Probiotic A microbe thought to be beneficial to the host organism and is similar to beneficial microorganisms found in the human gut. Probiotics are available to consumers mainly in the form of foods such as in yogurt or as dietary supplements.

Propolis Also known as bee's glue, a waxy resin produced by honeybees from the buds of trees as cement for their hives. It is used as an antibiotic and fungicide found in bio-cosmetics, face creams, ointments, lotions, solutions, varnishes, toothpastes, mouth-washes, tablets and chewing gums.

Propylene glycol An organic compound frequently used as a solvent, softening agent, moisturizer, preservative or vehicle in various personal products, medications, and industry. Propylene glycol may cause systemic contact dermatitis

Protease An enzyme that catalyzes the hydrolysis of proteins into peptide fractions and amino acids.

Rubber accelerators Chemicals that increases the speed of curing of rubber used in the manufacture of both natural latex and synthetic rubbers. Many of these agents can cause allergic dermatitis include thiurams, carbamates, mixed dialkyl thioureas and benzothiazoles. They may also be found in pesticides, some soaps and shampoos as bacteriostatic agents, adhesives, and elastic.

Quaternium-15 Quaternium-15 is commonly used in personal care products such as cosmetics, soaps and shampoos, and industrial substances. Quaternium-15 releases free formaldehyde and contact allergy can be due to the parent molecule itself or to formaldehyde.

Sensitization An immunologic state or condition in which previously encountered foreign substance triggers an immune reaction which may be antibody-mediated, particularly IgE, or cell-mediated. Subsequent exposure to the same antigen elicits an allergic response.

Sesquiterpene lactone A chemical compound found in the oleoresin fraction of leaf, stem, flower and possibly in the pollen of many plants in a group commonly known as *Compositae*. Sesquiterpene lactone can cause allergic reactions from Compositae contact allergy.

Sodium lauryl sulfate A surfactant commonly used in many personal care products such as toothpastes, soaps, shampoos and shaving creams. Although Sodium lauryl sulfate is considered safe at the concentrations used in cosmetic products, it can be an irritant similar to other detergents, with the irritation increasing with concentration.

Superantigen A powerful antigen occurring in various bacteria and viruses that binds outside of the normal T cell receptor site, reacting with multiple T cell receptor molecules and activating a large number of activated T-cells resulting in a massive immune response of T cells nonspecifically. Superantigens play an important role in some diseases including Staphylococcal toxic shock syndrome, Staphylococcal scalded skin syndrome and atopic dermatitis. Staphylococcal superantigens appear to be one of the important triggering factors that contribute to the cutaneous inflammation in atopic dermatitis.

Substance P A neuropeptide released from the terminals of specific sensory nerves. It is associated with inflammatory processes and pain. It functions as a neurotransmitter especially in the transmission of pain impulses from peripheral receptors to the central nervous system.

Th1 A subset of T-helper lymphocytes which synthesize and secrete interleukin-2, gamma-interferon, and interleukin-12. Th1 cytokines are associated with delayed-type hypersensitivity reactions.

Th2 A subset of T-helper lymphocytes which synthesize and secrete IL-4, IL-5, IL-6, and IL-10. These cytokines stimulate B-cell development and antibody production. The Th2 cytokines counteract the effects of the Th1 cytokines and can produce an anti-inflammatory response in the setting of Th1 activation

T regulatory cells A subpopulation of T cells that down-regulate the immune system, maintaining the ability to not attack an antigen that is part of the body itself (tolerance to self-antigens), and suppresses autoimmune disease. There are several different types of regulatory T cells.

Tixocortal pivalate A topical corticosteroid and also a screening marker for contact allergies to group A steroids including hydrocortisone and Prednisone

Tolerance An immunological state characterized by decreased responsiveness to an antigen that normally produces an immunological reaction.

Urticarial Relating to or marked by urticaria which is also called hives, an extremely itchy skin condition characterized by transient appearance of raised, well-circumscribed areas of edema and erythema (wheals and flares) involving the dermis and epidermis. The causes may include an allergic reaction, infection, or emotional stress.

Index

S.T. Nedorost, *Generalized Dermatitis in Clinical Practice*,   147
DOI 10.1007/978-1-4471-2897-7,
© Springer-Verlag London 2012